# Bath Salts and Other Synthetic Drugs

Drugs

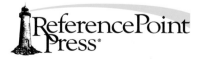

ReferencePoint
Press®

San Diego, CA

## Other books in the Compact Research Drugs set:

Club Drugs
Cocaine and Crack
Diet Drugs
Hallucinogens
Heroin
Methamphetamine
Oxycodone
Painkillers
Prescription Drugs

*For a complete list of titles please visit www.referencepointpress.com.

COMPACT *Research*

# Bath Salts and Other Synthetic Drugs

Peggy J. Parks

Drugs

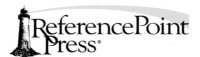

ReferencePoint Press®

San Diego, CA

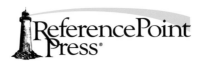

© 2014 ReferencePoint Press, Inc.
Printed in the United States

**For more information, contact:**
ReferencePoint Press, Inc.
PO Box 27779
San Diego, CA 92198
www.ReferencePointPress.com

Picture credits:
Cover: iStockphoto.com
Maury Aaseng: 33–35, 47–49, 61–63, 75–76
AP Images: 16
© Mills, Andy/Star Ledger/Corbis: 12

LIBRARY OF CONGRESS CATALOGING-IN-PUBLICATION DATA

Parks, Peggy J., 1951–
    Bath salts and other synthetic drugs / by Peggy J. Parks.
       pages cm. -- (Compact research series)
    Includes bibliographical references and index.
    ISBN-13: 978-1-60152-516-1 (hardback) -- ISBN-10: 1-60152-516-8 (hardback)
  1. Designer drugs. 2. Synthetic drugs. 3. Drugs of abuse. I. Title.
    RM316.P37    2014
    362.29'9--dc23
                                                                            2013015820

# Contents

# Foreword

**66Where is the knowledge we have lost in information?99**

—T.S. Eliot, "The Rock."

As modern civilization continues to evolve, its ability to create, store, distribute, and access information expands exponentially. The explosion of information from all media continues to increase at a phenomenal rate. By 2020 some experts predict the worldwide information base will double every seventy-three days. While access to diverse sources of information and perspectives is paramount to any democratic society, information alone cannot help people gain knowledge and understanding. Information must be organized and presented clearly and succinctly in order to be understood. The challenge in the digital age becomes not the creation of information, but how best to sort, organize, enhance, and present information.

ReferencePoint Press developed the *Compact Research* series with this challenge of the information age in mind. More than any other subject area today, researching current issues can yield vast, diverse, and unqualified information that can be intimidating and overwhelming for even the most advanced and motivated researcher. The *Compact Research* series offers a compact, relevant, intelligent, and conveniently organized collection of information covering a variety of current topics ranging from illegal immigration and deforestation to diseases such as anorexia and meningitis.

The series focuses on three types of information: objective single-author narratives, opinion-based primary source quotations, and facts and statistics. The clearly written objective narratives provide context and reliable background information. Primary source quotes are carefully selected and cited, exposing the reader to differing points of view, and facts and statistics sections aid the reader in evaluating perspectives. Presenting these key types of information creates a richer, more balanced learning experience.

For better understanding and convenience, the series enhances information by organizing it into narrower topics and adding design features that make it easy for a reader to identify desired content. For example, in *Compact Research: Illegal Immigration*, a chapter covering the economic impact of illegal immigration has an objective narrative explaining the various ways the economy is impacted, a balanced section of numerous primary source quotes on the topic, followed by facts and full-color illustrations to encourage evaluation of contrasting perspectives.

The ancient Roman philosopher Lucius Annaeus Seneca wrote, "It is quality rather than quantity that matters." More than just a collection of content, the *Compact Research* series is simply committed to creating, finding, organizing, and presenting the most relevant and appropriate amount of information on a current topic in a user-friendly style that invites, intrigues, and fosters understanding.

# Bath Salts and Other Synthetic Drugs at a Glance

## Synthetic Drugs Defined

Synthetic drugs are substances that are made entirely from chemicals, which distinguishes them from plant-based drugs such as cocaine, heroin, and marijuana.

## Types of Synthetic Drugs

The three main categories of synthetic drugs are stimulants (bath salts), relaxants (synthetic cannabinoids), and hallucinogens.

## Availability

People have purchased synthetic drugs at head shops, convenience stores, gas stations, tobacco shops, adult novelty stores, and on the Internet.

## Fraudulent Marketing

Synthetic drugs are called by a variety of names (such as "bath salts") that have nothing to do with what the substances are, and they are deceptively labeled "Not for human consumption."

## Seriousness of Problem

Based on calls to poison control centers throughout the United States, synthetic drug prevalence has increased significantly in only a few years.

## Dangers

Synthetic drugs have been associated with severe psychosis, suicidal thoughts and attempts, damage to vital organs, heart attacks, irreversible brain damage, and death.

## Regulation

Numerous substances used to make synthetic drugs have been banned through federal and state laws. This is a challenging issue, however, as underground chemists simply create new drugs with slightly different formulas.

## Treatment

There are no treatments specifically for synthetic drugs, since they have not been around long enough; typically, treatment regimens are based on other types of drug abuse and addiction.

## Prevention

Health officials stress that the key to preventing synthetic drug abuse is education and awareness; antidrug organizations, schools, and communities are working to develop prevention programs.

# Overview

The stories sound more like something out of a horror movie than actual news. A man in Tampa, Florida, runs into a busy intersection shouting, singing, and beating on car windows, and later dies of a drug overdose. A woman in Utica, New York, lunges at a police officer and tries to bite his face, screaming that she wants to "kill someone and eat them."[1] A West Virginia man, dressed in women's lingerie, steals his neighbor's pygmy goat and stabs it to death. A growling, snapping man from Miami, Florida, snarls at police officers and tries to bite them after being arrested for fighting. A man and woman in West Pittston, Pennsylvania, have become convinced that ninety people are living inside their walls. When police officers arrive at their apartment they find the couple frantically ripping down drywall, sticking their heads into the holes, and stabbing at the "intruders" with large knives.

As far-fetched as these accounts may seem, they are not fiction; each was a case investigated by law enforcement during 2011 or 2012. The people involved were from different areas of the country, but they shared one thing in common: All were high on synthetic drugs that are colloquially known as "bath salts." Packets of these drugs are sold under a wide variety of names, including Cloud 9, Bliss, Ivory Wave, Vanilla Sky, Red Dove, White Dove, and Cosmic Blast. But, says the National Institute on Drug Abuse (NIDA), "Don't let the fun names fool you. Bath salts are extremely dangerous."[2]

## What Are Synthetic Drugs?

The word "synthetic" means the opposite of "natural." A synthetic object is created by humans rather than by nature, so synthetic drugs are those that are made (synthesized) entirely from chemicals. This trait distinguishes synthetic drugs from those that are made from plants, such as marijuana, which comes from the *Cannabis sativa* plant; cocaine, which is made from the coca plant; and heroin, which is made from opium poppies. In a September 2012 presentation, the Substance Abuse and Mental Health Services Administration (SAMHSA) writes: "Synthetic drugs are chemical creations that are made to cause the same changes in the user's body as illegal drugs derived from plants."[3]

> " Bath salts are stimulant drugs, which are so-named because they stimulate (excite) the central nervous system. "

Synthetic drugs (sometimes called designer drugs) are categorized into three main groups: stimulants, relaxants, and hallucinogens. Although each has its own unique characteristics, a common trait is that they all have psychoactive properties. Psychoactive drugs are those that are capable of altering brain function, leading to temporary changes in perception, mood, consciousness, and behavior.

## From Bath Salts to "Smiles"

Bath salts are stimulant drugs, which are so-named because they stimulate (excite) the central nervous system. No one knows exactly where

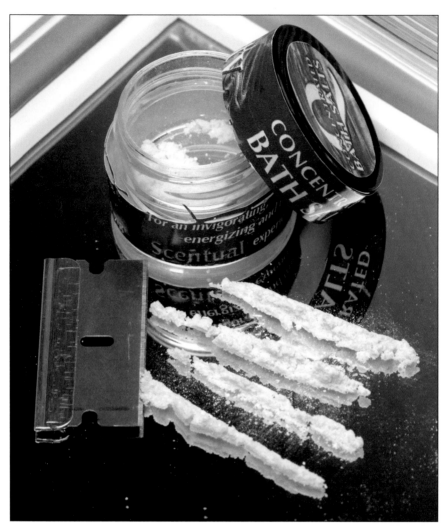

*Shown here is a 500 mg jar of "bath salts." The origin of the term bath salts is unknown although experts say it is clearly an attempt to disguise the true nature of the substances, which act as stimulants on the central nervous system.*

the term "bath salts" originated, although it was obviously an attempt at camouflaging the true nature of the substances. Bath salts are synthetic versions of cathinone, an organic stimulant that comes from the *Catha edulis* plant, better known as khat. This flowering shrub is native to East Africa and the Arabian Peninsula, and for centuries its leaves have been chewed or brewed in tea to produce an amphetamine-like high.

The synthetic cathinones in bath salts have complex-sounding names such as mephedrone, methylone, and methylenedioxypyrovalerone (MDPV). These drugs are usually in the form of a white or beige-colored powder that may be inhaled (snorted), smoked, or ingested with food or drinks. Some people liquefy the drugs over heat and inject them into a vein.

Smokeable synthetic drugs that are designed to mimic the effects of marijuana are sold under names such as K2, Spice, Blaze, and Black Mamba. These contain synthetic cannabinoids, which are chemical versions of the psychoactive ingredient in marijuana, tetrahydrocannabinol (THC)—but according to the National Association of Boards of Pharmacy, synthetic cannabinoids can be up to five hundred times stronger than THC. Often referred to as "fake weed" or "fake pot," synthetic marijuana consists of dried, shredded plant material that has been sprayed with a mixture of chemicals. These substances may look like potpourri or be ground into a powder that has the texture and color of oregano.

> " With billions of websites currently online, it is impossible for law enforcement to keep track of them all, even if the substances being sold are illegal. "

Synthetic hallucinogens are created to mimic the effects of psychedelic drugs such as LSD—but are far more potent. One example is the 2C family of drugs, such as 2C-E ("Europa") and 2C-I ("Smiles"), which are often said to be more powerful than a combination of MDMA (ecstasy) and LSD. People who have used these drugs typically report an intense high along with auditory and visual hallucinations that sometimes last for days.

## How People Get Synthetic Drugs

Before 2011, when state and federal law enforcement authorities began clamping down on synthetic drug sellers, the drugs were easy for almost anyone to get. People could buy them at "head shops" (stores that sell drug paraphernalia), convenience stores, smoke shops, adult novelty stores, and gas stations, as well as order them online. "Our biggest problem to start with was this stuff was easier to buy than bubble gum," says Palm Beach County, Florida, sheriff Ric Bradshaw. "It was in the gas stations, the convenience stores. The proliferation was unbelievable."[4]

> " Every time users take a synthetic drug, they are putting chemicals into their bodies without having the slightest idea what those chemicals are. "

Buying synthetic drugs has become more challenging in recent years, but users can still find them without too much trouble. Seventeen-year-old Max Earney, who lives in Broward County, Florida, no longer uses synthetic marijuana but says that if he wanted some, he knows exactly where to go. A clerk at one particular store where he used to buy Spice will pull out a hidden box and sell him the latest brands. "They don't even ask for ID," says Earney. "But they'll only sell it to you if they trust you."[5] One of the leading sources of synthetic drugs is the Internet. With billions of websites currently online, it is impossible for law enforcement to keep track of them all, even if the substances being sold are illegal.

## The Story Behind Synthetic Drugs

Although synthetic drugs have existed for decades, they were originally developed for research purposes only. During the 1970s medicinal chemist Richard A. Glennon created a synthetic version of cathinone while experimenting with stimulants and hallucinogens. Glennon's purpose was to evaluate how the substances affected the brain. About two decades later, organic chemist John W. Huffman synthesized cannabinoids to also be used for brain research. Neither Huffman nor Glennon ever intended for their chemical formulas to be used to make synthetic drugs for human use—but that is what happened.

According to the European Monitoring Centre for Drugs and Drug Addiction, smokeable herbal mixtures under the brand name Spice have been sold on the Internet and in various specialty shops since at least 2006. In the United States authorities discovered the country's first known batch of synthetic drugs in 2008. According to the Drug Enforcement Administration (DEA), in December of that year a massive shipment of Spice was seized and analyzed by US Customs and Border Patrol in Dayton, Ohio. Before long the DEA became aware that synthetic marijuana was making its way into the country and growing in popularity.

No one knows for sure exactly when bath salts made their first appearance in the United States. The substances initially came to the attention of the American Association of Poison Control Centers (AAPCC) in the autumn of 2010. The AAPCC became aware that people were arriving at hospital emergency rooms with serious, sometimes life-threatening reactions after using bath salts. Health care providers were not familiar with the substances and not sure what they were up against, so they contacted poison control centers.

## Dangerous Mysteries

When people use synthetic drugs, they are flirting with danger. There is no way for them to know which country the drugs came from, who made them, or under what kind of conditions they were produced—be it a filthy warehouse or a rat-infested garage. "They are completely invented and manufactured without any regulation, without any quality control, with nothing,"[6] says Phil Mendelson, who is chairman of the Committee on the Judiciary in Washington, DC.

Along with being in the dark about where and by whom synthetic drugs are made, buyers have no way of knowing what is in them. Reading a label is futile because if ingredient lists are there at all, they are deliberately incomplete or fraudulent. Tests performed on synthetic marijuana called Banana Cream Nuke detected fifteen different cannabinoids but none of the ingredients were listed on the label. What this means is that every time users take a synthetic drug, they are putting chemicals into their bodies without having the slightest idea what those chemicals are. "At least with a natural ingredient, you know what it is," says Mendelson. "Whereas with synthetics you have not a clue what it is."[7]

## Effects of Synthetic Drugs

One of the most disturbing aspects of synthetic drug abuse is that these drugs have not been around long enough for much research to have been done on them. Says Matthew Johnson, a professor of behavioral pharmacology at Johns Hopkins University: "There is hardly any research at

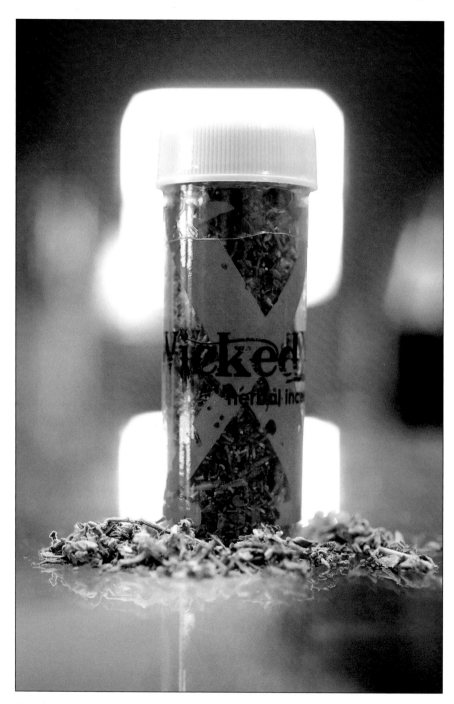

*Synthetic marijuana (pictured) is usually marketed as herbal incense and labeled as "Not for human consumption." Despite the label, people are smoking it to get high—and are experiencing dangerous side effects.*

all in the scientific literature on these things, even in animals, much less any sort of formal safety evaluation in humans."[8] Most of what is known about synthetic drugs has been gathered from user testimonials and reports from health care providers and law enforcement.

People who have taken bath salts have reportedly experienced everything from anxiety and agitation to confusion, painful headaches, nausea, and vomiting. A common side effect is bruxism, which is the habitual clenching of the jaw and grinding of the teeth. In the most severe cases, bath salts can cause irregular heartbeat, seizures, and psychosis, including frightening hallucinations.

> " Some people who smoke synthetic marijuana experience paranoia, auditory and visual hallucinations, delirium, and terrifying panic attacks. "

According to the military group Navy Alcohol and Drug Abuse Prevention, synthetic cannabinoids produce marijuana-like effects, including "euphoria, giddiness, silliness, bloodshot eyes, impaired short-term memory and concentration, and 'munchies.'"[9] Other common effects include sensitivity to light, "cotton mouth," dry eyes, and a warm sensation in the limbs. Some people who smoke synthetic marijuana experience paranoia, auditory and visual hallucinations, delirium, and terrifying panic attacks.

## How Serious a Problem Is Synthetic Drug Abuse?

Based on surveys conducted by agencies such as SAMHSA, the problem of synthetic drugs is nowhere near as serious as that of alcohol, marijuana, and some other drugs—yet. Without a doubt one of the most alarming aspects of synthetic drugs is how quickly their popularity has grown.

According to the AAPCC, which maintains the United States' only comprehensive poisoning surveillance database, the number of synthetic drug–related emergency calls to poison control centers began to spike in 2010. That year centers collectively reported about thirty-two hundred calls related to synthetic cannabinoids and bath salts—and by 2011 the number of calls had soared past thirteen thousand. Says DEA administrator Michele M. Leonhart: "In just one year, calls to Poison Control

Centers about synthetic cannabinoids such as Spice and K2 have more than doubled, and the calls regarding synthetic cathinones, marketed as bath salts, have increased more than 20 fold."[10]

At least 60 percent of the calls to poison control centers involved individuals under the age of twenty-five. This is consistent with what emergency room doctors and drug addiction experts are finding: that synthetic drug use is most prevalent among younger people. A 2011 study by the NIDA found that synthetic marijuana is the second most commonly abused drug among high school seniors after natural marijuana. The NIDA explains: "Easy access and the misperception that Spice products are 'natural' and therefore harmless have likely contributed to their popularity.

> As soon as drugs become illegal, unscrupulous chemists simply change a molecule or two and create new drugs to replace them.

Another selling point is that the chemicals used in Spice are not easily detected in standard drug tests."[11] Based on anecdotal evidence, bath salts appear to be favored more by young adults aged twenty to twenty-nine than by teens.

## What Are the Dangers of Synthetic Drugs?

Even though synthetic drugs have not been around that long, physicians and health officials already know that the substances are dangerous in many ways. Because drugs are absorbed into the bloodstream and carried throughout the body, they can affect all the major organs. Like any drug, synthetic drugs can cause an immediate toxicity reaction as the body tries to excrete them through vomiting, diarrhea, or sweating. This can lead to liver and kidney failure as the organs futilely attempt to filter toxins out of the body. The body's reaction to the synthetic drugs can also cause problems with the circulatory and nervous systems, leading to increased blood pressure and heart attacks.

By far the most dangerous risk associated with synthetic drugs is their effects on the brain. Users take the drugs to get high—and any drug that has the ability to make someone high does so by acting on the brain.

Cynthia R. Lewis-Younger, who is managing and medical director for the Florida Poison Information Center in Tampa, explains: "Because people take them for their psychological effects, they all go into the brain. We know that drug use can change the brain. Particularly with the synthetic cathinones, we've been seeing severe outcomes [including psychotic behaviors]. We don't know if those are permanent, but I think it will be likely. We have seen seizures and very high temperatures, both of which can be deadly."[12]

## How Should Synthetic Drugs Be Regulated?

The DEA continuously collects and reviews scientific, medical, and law enforcement data about emerging drugs of concern. Once these drugs have been identified, the US Congress has the power to ban them by listing each drug by name in legislation or by giving regulators the power to add the drugs to lists of controlled substances. In the United States, the term "controlled substances" refers to drugs that are listed in the Controlled Substances Act, which was originally passed in 1971 and has been amended a number of times since.

Controlled substances are organized into schedules, meaning lists of drugs to which special regulations apply. Substances are listed on one of five schedules based on factors such as therapeutic value, potential for abuse, and likelihood of causing addiction. Schedule I drugs, for instance, are those that the federal government deems to have no medically accepted use, are not considered safe even with medical supervision, and have high potential for abuse. Thus, the drugs are illegal except for research purposes.

In accordance with the Synthetic Drug Abuse Prevention Act of 2012, fifteen synthetic cannabinoids, two synthetic cathinones, and nine hallucinogenic drugs in the 2C family are now listed as Schedule I substances. As the DEA identifies additional substances of concern, others will undoubtedly be added to Schedule I. This pres-

> "Because synthetic drugs have not been around for a long period of time, public awareness of these drugs is low—and experts say that needs to change.

ents an ongoing challenge for the DEA and legislators; as soon as drugs become illegal, unscrupulous chemists simply change a molecule or two and create new drugs to replace them. Says Peter Delany, director of SAMHSA's Center for Behavioral Health Statistics and Quality: "You can ban chemicals, but if manufacturers modify the chemical format, they are no longer on the banned list."[13]

## Treatment Challenges

Although numerous substance abuse treatment programs exist throughout the United States, few if any are aimed specifically at synthetic drug use. These drugs are new to health care providers, and treatments are still evolving. Typically, people first seek help at emergency rooms after having a bad reaction to the drugs. Medical personnel must first calm the person down, keep him or her as comfortable and safe as possible, and possibly use medications to help with symptoms. Once the patient has been stabilized and is no longer in immediate danger, a physician will determine whether further treatment is warranted and make recommendations accordingly.

When people are treated for synthetic drug abuse, their treatment regimen is similar to that used for addiction to other types of drugs. It typically involves a team of professionals including physicians, mental health therapists, and social workers who are knowledgeable about community resources. In tandem with a treatment program patients are often encouraged to participate in twelve-step substance abuse programs such as those used by Alcoholics Anonymous and Narcotics Anonymous.

## How Can Synthetic Drug Abuse Be Prevented?

Because synthetic drugs have not been around for a long period of time, public awareness of these drugs is low—and experts say that needs to change. Kristin Wenger, who is a health educator at the Blue Ridge Poison Center at the University of Virginia School of Medicine, regularly encounters this lack of awareness. "When I go out and talk to groups of people," says Wenger, "I find that lots of people have heard of 'bath salts,' but they're not very sure what they are. A lot of them are still confused. They still think they are the actual bath salts you pour right into your tub, and that some odd person decided to start snorting them. That's not what they are at all."[14]

It is an established fact that the key to increasing awareness is education. To broaden young people's understanding of how dangerous synthetic drugs are, schools throughout the United States are adding information about the drugs to their existing drug awareness programs. Advocacy groups are conducting media campaigns to try to raise awareness about the dangers of synthetic drug use. Groups such as SAMHSA and NIDA have added sections to their websites to educate the public about what synthetic drugs are and the dangers involved with them. At the Partnership at Drugfree.org, social workers who are certified substance abuse counselors staff a parents' help line. Their goal is to increase parental awareness of synthetic drug use while building an online support community.

## "In the Shadows"

Health officials, physicians, and addiction experts view synthetic drugs as one of the most challenging, frightening issues they have ever encountered. These drugs are being widely abused, most often by young people, even though so much about the drugs is unknown. No one knows where they come from, who makes them, or exactly what they contain. In an effort to stop the proliferation of synthetic drugs, Congress has enacted legislation—but as soon as laws are passed, drug producers find ways around them. Physician Zane Horowitz, medical director of the Oregon Poison Center, shares his thoughts: "Unfortunately, the law won't make this problem disappear. We're going to continue to see a lot of this type of thing. It will always be in the shadows."[15]

# How Serious a Problem Is Synthetic Drug Abuse?

66Reports of severe intoxication and dangerous health effects associated with use of bath salts have made these drugs a serious and growing public health and safety issue.99

—National Institute on Drug Abuse, which seeks to end drug abuse and addiction in the United States.

66Over the past couple of years, smokeable herbal products marketed as being 'legal' and as providing a marijuana-like high, have become increasingly popular, particularly among teens and young adults.99

—Drug Enforcement Administration, the top federal drug law enforcement agency in the United States.

During his long, prestigious career as an organic chemist, John W. Huffman conducted extensive scientific research on the brain and nervous system. Beginning in 1984 he and his student assistants at Clemson University created hundreds of synthetic compounds, most of which were designated by the letters "JWH" (Huffman's initials) followed by numbers. A primary focus of this research was to study the interaction between the drugs and brain receptors. These are proteins that recognize specific chemicals in the brain and facilitate transmission of rapid-fire messages to and from nerve cells known as neurons.

In tests with laboratory animals some of Huffman's compounds have shown promise for development of chronic pain treatments. Others could potentially lead to treatments for inflammation as well as some types of skin cancer. These and other noted accomplishments are Huffman's true legacy as a scientist—but as the inventor of synthetic cannabinoids, he has also been the target of unwarranted blame and criticism.

Huffman's compounds were developed solely for research purposes and were never meant for use by humans. But that did not stop unscrupulous chemists from plucking the formulas out of scientific journals and using them to make and sell synthetic versions of marijuana. "He was doing good research," says Mark Ryan, director of the Louisiana Poison Control Center. "He never intended for his compounds to end up on the street."[16]

## "Russian Roulette"

Huffman's synthetic cannabinoid research began in 1984, supported by a generous grant from the National Institutes of Health. It is well known that when people smoke marijuana, the THC in the drug switches on the brain's cannabinoid receptors, which are involved with a number of mental and physical processes. "These receptors don't exist so that people can smoke marijuana and get high," says Huffman. "They play a role in regulating appetite, nausea, mood, pain and inflammation."[17] Huffman thought that if he could create a synthetic compound that flipped the receptor switch more effectively than THC, scientists could use the compound as a tool to unlock some of the brain's many secrets.

Huffman first became aware that his research had been exploited in December 2008, when someone forwarded an article to him from the German magazine *Der Spiegel.*

> " Although synthetic cannabinoids are structurally different from THC, they have nearly identical biological effects on the human body, which is why they are useful in research. "

The article described how mixtures of herbs, laced with the synthetic cannabinoid JWH-018, were being marketed and sold as a substitute for marijuana. Huffman had published his research in a 1998 article in the *Journal of Pharmacology & Experimental Therapeutics*. A longer, more involved paper on JWH-018 appeared in a 2005 article in the *Journal of Bioorganic and Medicinal Chemistry*. Huffman has no way of knowing who used his compounds to create synthetic marijuana, but he is not really surprised that someone did. "These people are not naive," he says. "They thought, 'Ah-ha! Let's try this stuff and smoke it.' . . . It's pretty simple to make if you have an organic chemistry lab."[18]

> " The speed at which bath salts abuse grew in the United States was astounding. "

Although synthetic cannabinoids are structurally different from THC, they have nearly identical biological effects on the human body, which is why they are useful in research. But some of the compounds, like JWH-018, are five to ten times stronger than THC, and scientists cannot predict how they might affect the brain over the long term. Huffman says that some of his more complex compounds are even more potent than JWH-018—meaning that they can have "profound psychological effects" and carry a risk for severe psychosis. "These things are dangerous," says Huffman. "Anybody who uses them is playing Russian roulette."[19]

## A Crisis Emerges

Synthetic marijuana had been in circulation for close to two years when US health officials started hearing about bath salts. During the late fall of 2010 the AAPCC became aware of a growing problem with the substances. Some of its member centers were receiving emergency phone calls about people having serious, sometimes life-threatening reactions after taking bath salts. Says AAPCC president Rick Dart: "Poison control experts were the first to raise the alarm about the products."[20]

The speed at which bath salts abuse grew in the United States was astounding. According to AAPCC data, the number of bath salts–related calls jumped from fourteen in August 2010 to nearly two hundred in December. One of the first states to be hit by the bath salts crisis was Louisiana, as raw ingredients were being shipped to the Port of New Orleans from China. "It came on like a freight train," says Ryan. From emergency department personnel he learned that people high on the drugs were suffering from worse hallucinations than those who took LSD. He was also told that overall, bath salts users were experiencing effects more severe than those produced by other drugs. Says Ryan: "It's not like it's just a bad drug. It's like a superbad drug."[21]

AAPCC data present a clear picture of the rapid growth of bath salts from the time the substances were first detected in the United States. During 2010 the agency recorded 304 bath salts–related calls. From that point on the number steadily grew, and by the end of 2011 calls about bath salts had ballooned to 6,136. This trend continued into 2012 with a rise in calls each month from January through June.

Then, according to the AAPCC, the crisis showed signs of abating. By the end of 2012 the number of bath salts–related calls nationwide totaled 2,655, which was a 57 percent decline from 2011. Some people speculated that this resulted from the combination of increased awareness and tougher legislation. According to Ryan, however, a more likely explanation is that as emergency room personnel became more accustomed to seeing bath salts cases, they no longer felt the need to call poison control centers.

## Shady Marketing

In an effort to promote their products, makers of synthetic drugs have used a number of unscrupulous tactics that Harvard Medical School psychiatry professor Bertha K. Madras refers to as "devious, aggressive marketing schemes."[22] The name "bath salts" is a prime example, since the drugs inside the packages have nothing to do with bathing. As awareness of bath salts has grown, producers have increasingly begun using different product names on labels, such as plant food, jewelry cleaner, insect repellant, and research chemicals. Similarly, producers of synthetic marijuana often label their packages as incense or potpourri. To further the deception, synthetic drugs are almost always labeled "Not for human consumption" as a tactic for skirting legal regulation and avoiding prosecution.

Some types of synthetic drugs are marketed to children in packages designed to look like they contain candy. These drugs have names that appeal to kids, such as Cotton Candy and Scooby Snax. The latter are sealed inside glossy packets with cartoon pictures of a dazed-looking Scooby Doo on the front. Affixed to the packets are stickers that say the contents are blueberry flavored, as though they were candy rather than drug-laced plant material. In Baltimore, Maryland, minister and activist Cortly "C.D." Witherspoon has been on a mission to keep these drugs out of the hands of the city's youth. He and his brother scope out convenience stores that sell Scooby Snax and report the businesses to law enforcement. Witherspoon, who is head of the local chapter of the Southern Christian Leadership Conference, says he considers any business, however otherwise legitimate, that sells synthetic drugs to be the equivalent of "a drug pusher."[23]

> " As awareness of bath salts has grown, producers have increasingly begun using different product names on labels, such as plant food, jewelry cleaner, insect repellant, and research chemicals. "

Synthetic drugs are increasingly being marketed on the Internet. Encouraged by drug manufacturers, users have built online communities where they can connect with each other to compare experiences. Some have brazenly shared homemade tutorial videos that explain how to make or use drugs. Says Tom Hedrick, founder and senior program officer of the Partnership at Drugfree.org: "Synthetic drug users share their highs and other experiences online, and these websites then allow an accelerated learning curve related to synthetic drug use, a 'how-to guide' for teens and young adults."[24] Technically, no one under the age of eighteen should be able to access websites that sell drugs, but site administrators have no way to verify the age of customers.

## Teen Trends

Although there has been a great deal of publicity about synthetic drugs, little substantive data exist about how widely they are being used. The authors of a report titled *Monitoring the Future* explain: "There has been very little scientific information about the prevalence of their use."[25] The report is the compilation of data from a major survey that was published in February 2013. It was conducted by a team of researchers from the University of Michigan and involved 45,400 students in eighth, tenth, and twelfth grade at 395 secondary schools throughout the United States. Although the survey has been conducted every year since 1975, this was the first time eighth and tenth graders were asked questions about synthetic marijuana, and the first time any questions were asked about bath salts.

One finding of the survey was that the marketing of synthetic drugs has influenced teen attitudes toward the use of Spice. Students in all three grades were asked whether they associated great risk with trying the drug once or twice, and less than one-fourth of them said they did. The report authors write: "Likely the availability of these drugs over the counter has communicated to teens that they must be safe, though they are not."[26]

The researchers found that 11.3 percent of twelfth graders had used synthetic marijuana sometime in the past twelve months. Among eighth graders, 4.4 percent said they had used the drug in the past year,

> **Although there has been a great deal of publicity about synthetic drugs, little substantive data exist about how widely they are being used.**

and exactly double that number (8.8 percent) of tenth graders said they had used it in the past year. Bath salts were much less common among teens. The survey found that 0.8 percent of eighth graders, 0.6 percent of tenth graders, and 1.3 percent of twelfth graders had used some kind of bath salts product in the past twelve months. "Fortunately," say the researchers, "we find the annual prevalence rates in 2012 to be very low."[27]

## A Guy Thing?

Although both males and females have been known to take synthetic drugs, these drugs are much more prevalent among teenage boys and young men. According to a December 2012 SAMHSA publication, nearly 80 percent of patients who made synthetic marijuana–related visits to emergency departments during 2010 were male. This has also been the trend with bath salts and other synthetic drugs, as Minnesota drug abuse strategy officer Carol L. Falkowski explains: "The primary users of these emerging synthetic drugs tend to be young males age 16 to 30, especially ones who are already in trouble with substance abuse, or the law, or both. For this group an added appeal of using these synthetic substances is that they are not routinely detected in standard urine screens."[28]

One teenage boy who became a habitual Spice user is Jake Suojanen, who is from the Tampa Bay area of Florida. After using the drug for about six months, Suojanen's grades plummeted from A's and B's to barely passing—but it was not his grades that caused him to stop smoking Spice. Rather, a seriously bad trip scared him into giving up the drug for good. In May 2012 Suojanen was smoking Spice with a friend's older brother and says the high was far more intense than he had ever experienced before. "My head was spinning and I couldn't see straight," he says. "I was pretty out of it."[29]

After inhaling the smoke deep into his lungs, Suojanen says, it was as if he could feel the world slipping away. He sat down on the edge of a bathtub and immediately blacked out. He has no memory of having seizures on the bathroom floor. He does not remember his friend yelling for someone to call 911. He does not remember riding to the hospital in an ambulance. Fortunately, doctors were able to save his life, and he made a full recovery. Suojanen is grateful to be alive—and has no intention of ever touching synthetic marijuana again.

## "Really Bad News"

Synthetic drugs have proved to be a formidable problem throughout the United States. Chemical compounds developed exclusively for research have been exploited for use in making synthetic marijuana. The prevalence of these drugs has soared since they were first created, as has the prevalence of bath salts—and this trend has health officials very concerned. Says Randy Badillo, clinical supervisor for Oklahoma's poison control center: "This stuff is really bad news."[30]

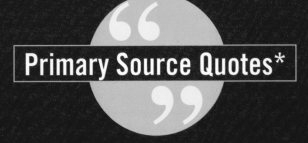

## How Serious a Problem Is Synthetic Drug Abuse?

**"Sold in legitimate-looking packaging, these insidious substances are marketed directly to teenagers and young adults with benign and catchy titles like Spice, Blaze, Vanilla Sky and incense."**

—Michele M. Leonhart, "*Operation Log Jam* Press Conference," July 26, 2012. www.justice.gov.

Leonhart is administrator of the Drug Enforcement Administration (DEA).

**"Think of these synthetic drugs . . . as ever-changing narcotic concoctions designed to be easily available and one step ahead of prosecution."**

— Indiana Prevention Resource Center, "Designer Drugs: A Wolf in Sheep's Clothing," June 26, 2012. www.drugs.indiana.edu.

The Indiana Prevention Resource Center works closely with Indiana-based alcohol, tobacco, and other drug prevention practitioners to improve the quality of their services.

* Editor's Note: While the definition of a primary source can be narrowly or broadly defined, for the purposes of Compact Research, a primary source consists of: 1) results of original research presented by an organization or researcher; 2) eyewitness accounts of events, personal experience, or work experience; 3) first-person editorials offering pundits' opinions; 4) government officials presenting political plans and/or policies; 5) representatives of organizations presenting testimony or policy.

❝Right behind Spice and Bath Salts, a whole line of synthetic or herbal products are emerging, many of which are being marketed along the same pathways and haven't been targeted yet by law enforcement.❞

—Brad Rollins and Mike Keleher, "Emerging Drug Trends," LawOfficer, September 24, 2012. www.lawofficer.com.

Rollins is an intelligence analyst with the Naval Criminal Investigative Service, and Keleher is division chief of Criminal Investigations, Violent Crime, and Cold Case Homicide with the same organization.

❝Products often are packaged with disingenuous labels such as 'not for human consumption' or 'incense,' but health professionals and legal authorities are keenly aware that these products are smoked like marijuana.❞

—Tracy D. Murphy et al., "Acute Kidney Injury Associated with Synthetic Cannabinoid Use—Multiple States, 2012," *Morbidity and Mortality Weekly Report*, Centers for Disease Control and Prevention, February 15, 2013. www.cdc.gov.

Murphy is a clinical pathologist from Cheyenne, Wyoming.

❝'Bath Salts' are manmade derivatives (i.e., synthetics) of naturally occurring stimulants, created and popularized by 'armchair chemists' driven by profit potential and whose business acumen is much more developed than their chemistry abilities.❞

—Hunterdon Drug Awareness Program, "Comprehensive Drug Information on Synthetic Cathinones—MDPV, Mephedrone & Methylone ('Bath Salts')," June 27, 2012. www.hdap.org.

Hunterdon Drug Awareness Program is a drug treatment facility located in Flemington, New Jersey.

❝ The internet has played a significant role in the explosion of synthetic drug use due to the ease of purchase and the difficulty in tracking such operations. ❞

—Council on Chemical Abuse, "Synthetic Drugs: Unstable & Dangerous," Fact Sheet, February 2, 2012. www.councilonchemicalabuse.org.

Located in Reading, Pennsylvania, the Council on Chemical Abuse serves as the coordinating agency for publicly supported programming against drug and alcohol abuse throughout the county.

❝ Bath Salt abuse has skyrocketed in recent years, largely due to the fact that these drugs had been, for the most part, legal. ❞

—Bonnie Nolan, "Are 'Bath Salts' Just Hype?," *Psychology Today*, October 3, 2012. www.psychologytoday.com.

Nolan is a neuroscientist and lecturer at Rutgers University.

❝ What makes this even trickier is that not all 'Bath Salts' are marketed as Bath Salts. Substituted cathinones and related drugs have been sold as plant feeder, insect repellent and even stain remover. ❞

—Partnership at DrugFree.org, "Synthetic Drugs: Bath Salts, K2/Spice: A Guide for Parents and Other Influencers," Parents 360, February 16, 2012. www.drugfree.org.

The Partnership at DrugFree.org is dedicated to helping parents and families solve the problem of teenage substance abuse.

❝ Exposure to and use of synthetic cathinones are increasingly popular despite a lack of scientific research and understanding of the potential harms of these substances. ❞

—Jane M. Prosser and Lewis S. Nelson, "The Toxicology of Bath Salts: A Review of Synthetic Cathinones," *Journal of Medical Toxicology*, March 2012. http://duienforcers.camp7.org.

Prosser and Nelson are emergency medicine physicians from New York City.

## How Serious a Problem Is Synthetic Drug Abuse?

- The American College of Emergency Physicians estimates that **60 percent** of synthetic drug users are under the age of twenty-five.

- According to a December 2012 report by the Substance Abuse and Mental Health Services Administration, synthetic cannabinoid drugs were linked to 11,406 of the **4.9 million** drug-related emergency department visits in 2010.

- A 2013 study of more than two thousand young adults conducted by Georgia Southern University professors John Stogner and Bryan Miller found that **14 percent** had used synthetic marijuana at some point in their lives.

- The American Association of Poison Control Centers reports receiving 2,906 **Spice-related calls** in 2010, and in 2011 the number rose to 6,955.

- According to a 2011 paper in the medical journal *Clinical Toxicology*, within eight months of their appearance in the United States, more than **fourteen hundred cases** of use and abuse of bath salts had been reported to poison centers in **forty-seven** of fifty states.

- According to the American Association of Poison Control Centers, there were more than six thousand bath salts–related calls **to poison control centers** during 2011, which was ten times the number reported in 2010.

# More Teens Abuse Synthetic Marijuana than Bath Salts

Health officials are concerned about the widespread abuse of synthetic drugs, especially by young people. During a 2012 survey called *Monitoring the Future*, students in eighth, tenth, and twelfth grades were asked questions about their use of a variety of substances, including synthetic drugs. As this graph shows, synthetic marijuana was shown to be much more common among teens of all grades than bath salts.

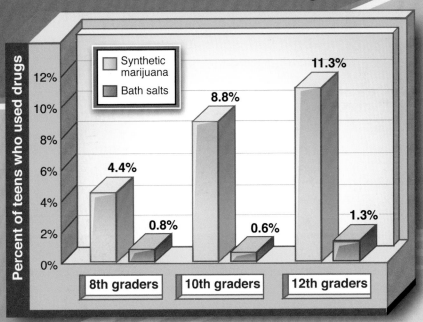

*Teens who used synthetic marijuana or bath salts sometime during 2012*

Source: Lloyd D. Johnston et al., *Monitoring the Future: National Results on Drug Use*, February 2013. www.monitoringthefuture.org.

- A December 2012 report by the Substance Abuse and Mental Health Services Administration revealed that the average age for people involved in **synthetic cannabinoid–related emergency department (ED) admissions** was younger than for marijuana-related ED visits (twenty-four years old versus thirty years old).

## Huge Spike in Bath Salts Use

The synthetic drugs known as bath salts were virtually unheard of in the United States prior to 2010. Then, during the late summer of that year, poison control centers in some of the southern states began receiving emergency calls about people having strange, sometimes violent reactions to the drugs. Before long, centers all over the country were receiving calls. This graph shows the huge spike in bath salts–related emergency calls between 2010 and 2011.

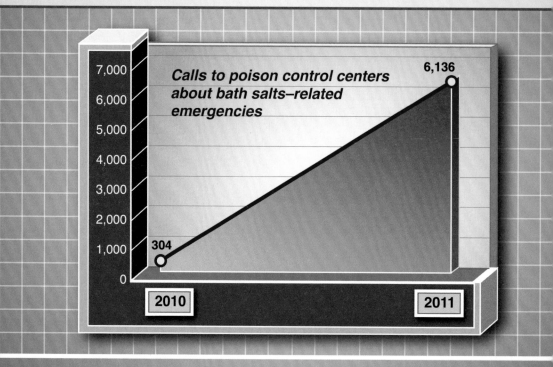

*Calls to poison control centers about bath salts–related emergencies*

304

6,136

2010

2011

Source: American Association of Poison Control Centers, "Bath Salts Data," March 31, 2013. https://aapcc.s3.amazonaws.com.

- Scientists at the Johnson County Crime Lab in Kansas City, Missouri, have found that **20 to 30 percent** of all drugs seized and tested in their laboratory are synthetic drugs.

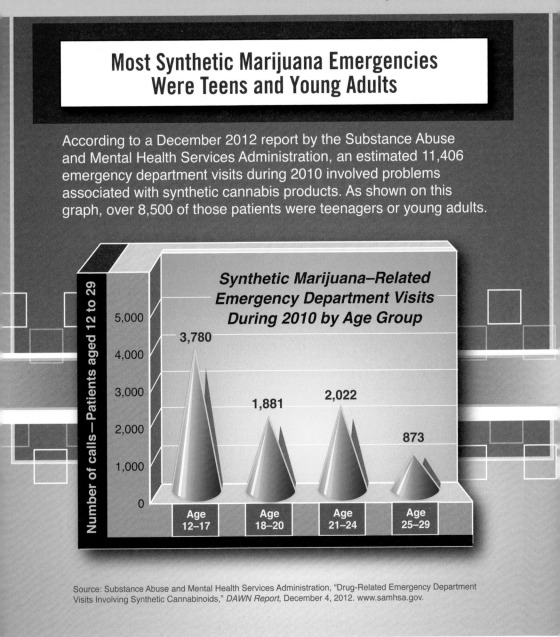

## Most Synthetic Marijuana Emergencies Were Teens and Young Adults

According to a December 2012 report by the Substance Abuse and Mental Health Services Administration, an estimated 11,406 emergency department visits during 2010 involved problems associated with synthetic cannabis products. As shown on this graph, over 8,500 of those patients were teenagers or young adults.

### Synthetic Marijuana–Related Emergency Department Visits During 2010 by Age Group

Number of calls—Patients aged 12 to 29

- Age 12–17: 3,780
- Age 18–20: 1,881
- Age 21–24: 2,022
- Age 25–29: 873

Source: Substance Abuse and Mental Health Services Administration, "Drug-Related Emergency Department Visits Involving Synthetic Cannabinoids," *DAWN Report*, December 4, 2012. www.samhsa.gov.

- In the 2012 *Monitoring the Future* survey, which was conducted by University of Michigan researchers and published in 2013, **4.4 percent** of eighth graders, **8.8 percent** of tenth graders, and **11.3 percent** of twelfth graders had used synthetic marijuana sometime during the past year.

# What Are the Dangers of Synthetic Drugs?

66Synthetic drugs can be extremely dangerous and addictive.99

—American Association of Poison Control Centers, which supports fifty-seven poison control centers throughout the United States and maintains the country's only comprehensive poisoning surveillance database.

66In addition to being highly addictive, 'bath salts' carry a significant risk for overdose.99

—Bonnie Nolan, a neuroscientist and lecturer at Rutgers University.

On the night of March 16, 2011, in the town of Blaine, Minnesota, seventeen-year-old Jesse Fisher was looking forward to hanging out with a couple of friends. His mom was out of town, so the teens went to a store that they knew would sell them beer, bought a thirty-pack, and took it back to Fisher's house. Two other kids dropped by, then a few more, and before long the small gathering had grown into a party.

At about 10:00 p.m. Fisher's friend Trevor Robinson showed up with Tim Lamere and two other friends. Soon after they arrived Lamere pulled a small bottle of grayish-white powder out of his pocket. He said it was a hallucinogenic 2C drug that he had legally bought online. After offering to share it with anyone who wanted some, Lamere poured the powder onto a table and split it into lines, and he and Robinson each snorted one. At first Fisher wanted nothing to do with the drug. Then he and most of the others ended up taking it too—and what happened was later described by police as a "mass overdose."[31]

## A Night of Terror and Tragedy

Everyone who used the drug felt its effects immediately, and the room erupted into chaos. People were holding their faces, crying out in pain, sweating, breathing heavily, and vomiting. Fisher, who calls it the "scariest experience" of his life, can hardly find the words to describe how bad the pain was. "It felt like I got kicked in the face by a horse," he says. "My brain felt like it was melting. It was so excruciating and painful, I couldn't even talk. All I could do is scream, grab my head and roll around on the floor."[32]

As much as Fisher suffered from the drug's effects, Robinson's reaction was worse. He began screaming and flailing his arms, erratically spinning around the room and punching holes in the walls. After a while he fell down and began having violent seizures—and then suddenly he quit breathing. His panicked friends administered CPR, but he did not respond. Two of them raced to the hospital with Robinson, carried him into the emergency room, and screamed for help. But doctors were not able to revive him, and he was pronounced dead that afternoon. Cause of death: cardiac arrest from 2C-E toxicity. Lamere was arrested and charged with unintentional third-degree murder and was later sentenced to ten years in prison.

> **Most users are unaware that the chemical composition of synthetic drugs can differ radically from one batch to the next.**

Robinson's friends were stunned and heartbroken over his death. "Why would he die out of all of us?" asks seventeen-year-old A.J. Carver, who was at the party and also took the drug. "We all did, like, the same amount. I don't know, it just freaks me out how any split second someone could be gone just because of a stupid decision."[33]

## Playing with Fire

No one can say for sure why the 2C-E killed Robinson and no one else. But the fact that young people take synthetic drugs at all is extremely disturbing to those who work in law enforcement and health care. So much about synthetic drugs is unknown, yet that does not stop people, most of whom are teens and young adults, from buying and using them without having any idea about where the drugs come from or what chemicals they contain. Says DEA agent Jeffrey Scott: "If I don't know as an investigator what's in those packets, how can anyone just buying them off the street or in those stores have any hope of knowing what's inside them—much less what it's going to do to them?"[34]

> **Laboratory tests on synthetic marijuana have also shown enormous inconsistencies from batch to batch.**

Most users are unaware that the chemical composition of synthetic drugs can differ radically from one batch to the next. Someone may use one of the 2C drugs, bath salts, or Spice without any problems—and have a horrible reaction the next time they use it. Because the drugs are produced without any regulation or quality control, no two packets are necessarily the same. Thus, there is a fine line between a mixture that can make someone feel euphoric and one that can cause permanent brain damage. A September 2012 PBS investigative report explains:

> It's the inconsistency of synthetic drugs that worries experts the most. Tiny mistakes in drugmakers' laboratories can make huge differences in how the drug reacts when it enters the human body. Simple highs can become debilitating illnesses. In 1982, in Northern California, for example, a synthetic heroin made in an underground lab caused a group of users to permanently develop symptoms nearly identical to advanced Parkinson's Disease.[35]

The dangerous inconsistencies of synthetic drugs have been highlighted in laboratory tests, such as those performed in 2010 at the Louisiana Poison Control Center. According to Mark Ryan, tests with bath salts found that one batch contained 17 milligrams of MDPV—and another batch of what was supposedly the same drug contained 2,000 milligrams of MDPV. Tests by law enforcement investigators in Arkansas found that bath salts contained at least 250 different chemicals.

Laboratory tests on synthetic marijuana have also shown enormous inconsistencies from batch to batch. Says NIDA scientist Marilyn A. Huestis: "You might buy a package one week, go back to the same place and buy the exact same package the next week, and the ingredients may be completely different. Not only are the ingredients unknown, but so is the strength of the drug." Huestis adds that because synthetic cannabinoids vary so much, studying the drugs is a major challenge, and the risks for anyone who uses them are immense. "Essentially," she says, "if you use it, you're experimenting on yourself."[36]

## Sinister Spice

People who smoke synthetic marijuana often say that they thought it was a legal and safe alternative to the real thing—and they were wrong on both counts. The drug has been associated with numerous health issues, some of which were life threatening. In March 2012, for instance, the Wyoming Department of Health became aware of three patients who were hospitalized for unexplained kidney damage. When the patients were interviewed for their medical history, all three admitted smoking synthetic marijuana. Health officials launched an investigation and found that the problem was not limited to Wyoming. A total of sixteen people in seven states were affected by unexplained kidney injuries. They ranged in age from fifteen to thirty-three, and all but one of the patients were male.

Although separated by hundreds of miles the cases were nearly identical. After smoking synthetic marijuana, each person was stricken with nausea, vomiting, and abdominal and/or back pain, and each went to a hospital emergency department. All sixteen were diagnosed with acute kidney injury, which doctors attributed to chemicals in synthetic marijuana that are toxic to the kidneys. "We knew that spice was dangerous," says Michael D. Schwartz of the National Center for Environmental Health's Office of Environmental Health Emergencies. "It's not a safe alternative to marijuana. As newer compounds come out in spice products, there is the risk of unpredictable toxicities."[37]

Health care professionals have also observed an association between synthetic marijuana and heart problems. Because smoking the drug speeds up heart rate and elevates blood pressure to dangerously high levels, the heart can be damaged. In 2010 three teenage boys from Dallas, Texas, learned this for themselves after they smoked synthetic marijuana. In cases unrelated to each other, the teens developed chest pains and were taken to the emergency department at Children's Medical Center Dallas. At the hospital, the chest pains grew more severe in two of the boys, and tests determined that they had suffered heart attacks—at the age of sixteen. Says physician Anthony Scalzo: "Youth and parents should be warned about the dangers of these substances. . . . You might be the next case report of a serious seizure, mental health crisis or perhaps a premature heart attack."[38]

## Severe, Lasting Psychosis

Medical professionals and health officials have learned that people high on synthetic drugs often act in ways that are bizarre and frightening. They show up at emergency rooms hyperagitated, burning with fever and dripping with sweat, and suffering from severe paranoia and hallucinations. According to Ryan, the patients are extremely difficult for medical personnel to handle. "For lack of a better term, they're flipped out," he says. "It's almost like a psychotic break. They're extremely anxious and combative, they think there's stuff trying to get them, they're paranoid, they're having hallucinations. So, the encounters are not pleasant." Ryan adds that some patients have been so psychotic that even large doses of sedatives could not calm them down: "We were finding that some of these guys couldn't be sedated with the normal drugs that we would use with other stimulants."[39]

> People who smoke synthetic marijuana often say that they thought it was a legal and safe alternative to the real thing—and they were wrong on both counts.

One particularly disturbing effect of bath salts is that the effects linger for a long time; some people still suffer from paranoia days or even weeks after they use the drugs. Scientists theorize that this lasting quality is due to the powerful stimulant MDPV, which is up to ten times stronger than cocaine. Although research is still in its infancy, scientists are learning that once MDPV latches onto brain cells, it clings to them like glue. "MDPV is irreversible, it won't let go," says Virginia Commonwealth University researcher Louis J. De Felice. "I don't know of any other drug that has that same feature of not allowing you to escape from it."[40] After snorting bath salts in November 2010, twenty-one-year-old Dickie Sanders could not escape from the drug's effects. He was gripped by intense, severe paranoia that held on for days—and it became so unbearable that he took his own life.

## From Cloud Nine to Suicide

Sanders had previously been in trouble with the law for marijuana abuse, but he was starting to get his life back on track. He was enrolled in a drug program, regularly attended group meetings, and underwent frequent drug testing as required. Then on November 10, 2010, a fellow group member offered him a white, powdery substance known as Cloud 9 bath salts. The man told Sanders that the drug would give him a great high with the added bonus of not showing up on drug tests. Sanders bought some, took it home, and snorted it—and almost immediately felt like he was descending into hell.

Sanders grew psychotic and desperate, plagued by terrifying hallucinations and delusions. He was certain that the police were hunting for him, and told his father to look outside because there were twenty-five patrol cars surrounding the property. Then, before anyone could stop him, Sanders grabbed a butcher knife and slashed his own throat. His father, a physician, grabbed him, put pressure on the wound, and was relieved to see that the blade had missed major arteries. He took Sanders to the hospital for treatment, where the young man admitted to using bath salts. After suturing his wound, doctors spent hours evaluating his mental health before releasing him. Over and over he said to his father, "I just want this stuff out of me."[41]

> **One particularly disturbing effect of bath salts is that the effects linger for a long time; some people still suffer from paranoia days or even weeks after they use the drugs.**

Sanders's hallucinations seemed to ease a little, and his father took him home, determined to stay with him for the night. Dr. Sanders wrapped his arms around his son and held him until the young man fell asleep. He did not hear his son get up and leave the room during the night, and when he woke up at 7:00 the next morning, he found that his son was not in bed. Dr. Sanders went looking and found his son on the floor of another room, blood pooling next to his head. The troubled young man had shot himself to death, and no one had heard the sound of the gun. Later, Dr. Sanders spoke about the substance that had led to his son's suicide: "This stuff is poison," he said. "You don't get high on it—you go crazy."[42]

## Ominous Substances

Even though synthetic drugs have been around for a relatively short period of time, they have proved to be unpredictable and dangerous. No one knows where the drugs come from or who produced them, and tests have shown huge inconsistencies even among the exact same types. The drugs have been associated with everything from extreme psychosis and long-lasting paranoia to heart attacks, kidney damage, and suicide. "You don't understand why someone would want to do this to themselves,"[43] says Ryan. Yet despite the enormous risks, synthetic drugs continue to be in demand—which means that lives continue to be at risk.

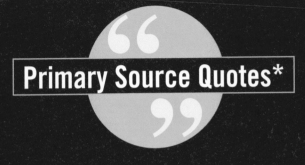

# What Are the Dangers of Synthetic Drugs?

66 **What makes synthetic marijuana so dangerous is that it is far more potent than cannabis and can lead to toxic, even fatal reactions.** 99

—Gregory Bunt, "Synthetic Marijuana: A New Clear and Present Danger," *Huffington Post*, February 22, 2012. www.huffingtonpost.com.

Bunt is medical director and senior vice president of Health Services at the New York residential treatment facility Daytop Village.

66 **According to some reports, the intoxication produced by synthetic cannabinoids is more intense than that produced by cannabis, while others report that it is milder.** 99

—Jenny L. Wiley, Julie A. Marusich, John W. Huffman, Robert L. Balster, and Brian F. Thomas, "Hijacking of Basic Research: The Case of Synthetic Cannabinoids," RTI International, November 2011. www.rti.org.

Wiley, Marusich, and Thomas are researchers with RTI International; Balster is director of the Institute for Drug and Alcohol Studies; and Huffman is a retired organic chemist who first created synthetic cannabinoids.

* Editor's Note: While the definition of a primary source can be narrowly or broadly defined, for the purposes of Compact Research, a primary source consists of: 1) results of original research presented by an organization or researcher; 2) eyewitness accounts of events, personal experience, or work experience; 3) first-person editorials offering pundits' opinions; 4) government officials presenting political plans and/or policies; 5) representatives of organizations presenting testimony or policy.

**❝Bath salts are among the most dangerous drugs a person can use.❞**

—Margaret Larson, "Recognizing Signs of Bath Salts," Global Good Group, August 28, 2012. http://globalgoodgroup.com.

Larson is a nurse and public health educator from Texas.

---

**❝Because the chemical composition of many products sold as Spice is unknown, it is likely that some varieties also contain substances that could cause dramatically different effects than the user might expect.❞**

—National Institute on Drug Abuse, "Spice (Synthetic Marijuana)," Drug Facts, December 2012. www.drugabuse.gov.

An agency of the National Institutes of Health, NIDA seeks to end drug abuse and addiction in the United States.

---

**❝Doctors and clinicians at U.S. poison centers have indicated that ingesting or snorting 'bath salts' containing synthetic stimulants can cause chest pains, increased blood pressure, increased heart rate, agitation, hallucinations, extreme paranoia, and delusions.❞**

—Nora Volkow, "'Bath Salts'—Emerging and Dangerous Products," National Institute on Drug Abuse, February 2011. www.drugabuse.gov.

Volkow is director of the NIDA.

---

**❝Synthetic drug abusers may endanger not only themselves but others: some become violent when under the influence of these substances, and abusers who operate motor vehicles after using synthetic drugs likely present similar dangers as those under the influence of controlled substances.❞**

—Ronald Weich, letter to the Honorable F. James Sensenbrenner Jr., September 30, 2011. www.justice.gov.

Weich is the assistant US attorney general.

---

66Numerous emergency department admissions have been connected to these substances, while law enforcement communications to DEA indicate multiple violent episodes linked to smoking these synthetic cannabinoids.99

—Drug Enforcement Administration, "Notice of Proposed Rulemaking," *Federal Register*, March 1, 2012. www.gpo.gov.

The DEA is the United States' top federal drug law enforcement agency.

66The effects of bath salts can be severe. Very severe paranoia can sometimes cause users to harm themselves or others.99

—Partnership at DrugFree.org, "Synthetic Drugs: Bath Salts, K2/Spice: A Guide for Parents and Other Influencers," Parents 360, February 16, 2012. www.drugfree.org.

The Partnership at DrugFree.org is dedicated to helping parents and families solve the problem of teenage substance abuse.

66Because of the spectrum of bath salts' effects, violent behavior can appear without warning.99

—Mark M. McGraw, "Is Your Patient High on 'Bath Salts'?," *Nursing*, January 2012. http://journals.lww.com.

McGraw is an emergency medicine nurse on the critical care transport team at Christiana Care Health Systems in Wilmington, Delaware.

66MDPV, Mephedrone, and other synthetic cathinones can cause serious psychiatric symptoms in people who have never exhibited such symptoms prior to usage.99

—Hunterdon Drug Awareness Program, "Comprehensive Drug Information on Synthetic Cathinones—MDPV, Mephedrone & Methylone ('Bath Salts')," June 27, 2012. www.hdap.org.

Hunterdon Drug Awareness Program is a drug treatment facility located in Flemington, New Jersey.

# What Are the Dangers of Synthetic Drugs?

- According to the Substance Abuse and Mental Health Services Administration, the synthetic cannabinoid known as **HU-210** is up to eight hundred times more potent than natural THC, the psychoactive chemical in marijuana.

- During a 2011 investigation Boston University School of Medicine psychiatrist Carlos Alverio determined that synthetic cannabis products such as **Spice** may pose a greater risk of psychosis than natural marijuana.

- According to the Partnership at DrugFree.org, users say that one of the most frightening effects of synthetic marijuana is **dysphoria**, which is an emotional state characterized by a deep sense of unhappiness.

- According to an April 2012 report by Cleveland Clinic physicians, of synthetic stimulant users who seek treatment at emergency rooms, 14 percent to 40 percent have **psychotic symptoms**.

- The Drug Enforcement Administration says that bath salts chemical **MDPV** has been reported to cause intense panic attacks, psychosis, and a strong desire to use the drug again.

- According to the National Institute on Drug Abuse, the bath salts chemical MDPV acts similar to cocaine in the way it affects brain chemicals but is **ten times more potent than cocaine**.

# The Many Dangers of Bath Salts

The drugs known as bath salts can cause a variety of problems ranging in severity from muscle tremors to severe panic attacks, seizures, and even death.

## Physical and Behavioral Effects of Bath Salts

| Physical Effects | Behavioral and Mental Effects |
|---|---|
| Tachycardia (abnormally fast heartbeat) | Panic attacks |
| Hypertension | Anxiety |
| Vasoconstriction (narrowing of blood vessels, which slows or blocks blood flow) | Agitation |
| Arrhythmias (abnormal heart rhythm) | Paranoia |
| Hyperthermia (abnormally high body temperature) | Hallucinations |
| Sweating | Psychosis |
| Mydriasis (prolonged, abnormally dilated pupils) | Aggressive behavior |
| Muscle tremor and spasms | Violent behavior |
| Seizures | Self-destructive behavior |
| Stroke | Self-mutilation |
| Cerebral edema (pressure on the skull due to excess fluid accumulation on the brain) | Suicidal thoughts |
| Respiratory distress | Insomnia |
| Cardiovascular collapse (sudden loss of blood flow to the heart) | Anorexia |
| Myocardial infarction (heart attack) | Depression |

## Synthetic Drugs Viewed as More Dangerous than Heroin and Cocaine

During a September 2012 survey of 1,021 people, participants were asked which substances they thought were the most dangerous for young people today. As this chart shows, synthetic drugs were viewed as more dangerous than marijuana, heroin, and cocaine, but less dangerous than methamphetamine, crack, or prescription painkillers.

### Which substance is the most dangerous for our kids in today's society?

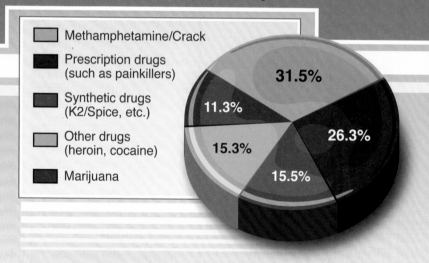

Methamphetamine/Crack

Prescription drugs
(such as painkillers)

Synthetic drugs
(K2/Spice, etc.)

Other drugs
(heroin, cocaine)

Marijuana

31.5%

11.3%

26.3%

15.3%

15.5%

Source: TestCountry, "TestCountry.com Survey Reveals Prescription Drugs & Synthetic Drugs Are Catching Up to Methamphetamine as the Most Dangerous Drug for Today's Teenagers," October 10, 2012. www.testcountry.com.

- According to a July 2012 report by public health physician Susan Cheng and colleagues, the number of reported **seizures** from synthetic cathinones in the United States increased from 14 in 2009 to 290 in 2010.

- The Partnership at DrugFree.org states that an especially troubling aspect of synthetic drugs is that there is no way to know how they might affect users in the **long term**.

# Why Bath Salts Are So Dangerous

Bath salts have only been in circulation in the United States since 2010, so researchers are only beginning to understand how the drugs affect the human brain. One expert is David Ferguson, who is professor and director of graduate studies at the University of Minnesota's School of Pharmacy. Shown on this diagram are some of the potential dangers of these drugs that Ferguson has identified.

## Risks of Bath Salts Use

| Risk | Explanation |
|------|-------------|
| Purity levels | Drugs are manufactured without regulatory guidelines and are likely to contain impurities. Chemical impurities often lead to extreme toxicities with long-term health effects for users. |
| Variable potency | Chemical compounds may vary drastically from product to product; a gram of one may be 50 to 100 times more potent than another. |
| Varying production guidelines | There are no official standards for making bath salts; recipes vary from batch to batch, and some manufacturers add fillers to expand quantity. These fillers can cause a negative and possibly deadly reaction in some users. |
| Issues for users of other drugs | For users accustomed to street drugs like cocaine, methamphetamine, or heroin, the reward/high is not as intense with bath salts; this can lead to higher usage and an increase in abuse/addiction potential, as well as lead to aggressive behaviors and severe health complications. |

Source: University of Minnesota, "As the Dangers of 'Bath Salts' Take Center Stage, U of M Researcher Explains the Dangerous Evolution of Synthetic Drugs," *Expert Alerts*, June 28, 2012.

- According to the American Association of Poison Control Centers, of the more than six thousand bath salts–related calls to US poison control centers in 2011, symptoms included **increased blood pressure, increased heart rate, agitation, hallucinations, extreme paranoia, and delusions.**

# How Should Synthetic Drugs Be Regulated?

66Unfortunately, despite legislation and bans, bath salts are still being used quite frequently.99

—Mark M. McGraw, an emergency medicine nurse on the critical care transport team at Christiana Care Health Systems in Wilmington, Delaware.

66Like synthetic cannabinoids . . . synthetic stimulants are very difficult to regulate because they are a large group of substances. As soon as one substance is outlawed, another synthetic stimulant will likely take its place.99

—Jason Jerry, Gregory Collins, and David Streem, physicians with Cleveland Clinic's Alcohol and Drug Recovery Center.

On December 25, 2010, Louisiana health officer Jimmy Guidry got a phone call from Mark Ryan at the state Poison Control Center. The center was usually quiet on Christmas Day, but not this year. Ryan was getting one call after another about emergencies that involved people who had taken bath salts—a total of eleven that morning. He knew that he was facing a crisis situation, so he canceled his holiday vacation plans and telephoned Guidry. "Merry Christmas," said Ryan. "I think you should know, my family's going skiing and I'm staying here."[44] Ryan explained that he could not leave because the center was in a state of emergency, and it required immediate action. He needed Guidry's help.

Guidry knew Ryan well and respected his professional opinion, so he immediately began to think about the best way of addressing the issue. He brought his legal team on board, had discussions with law enforcement professionals, and scrutinized the available data. It took only a week for Guidry to conclude that bath salts fit all the necessary criteria to be classified and controlled as dangerous substances. He called Ryan with the good news. "We're ready to move," said Guidry. "What should we ban?"[45] By January 6, 2011, Guidry had used what is known as "emergency rule," which gives state agency directors the authority to adopt rules that protect public health, safety, or welfare. The ban that Guidry enacted covered five of the most common synthetic cathinones found in bath salts.

## States Take Action

With Guidry's action, Louisiana became the first state to outlaw synthetic cathinones. Others began to pass their own laws, and by November 28, 2012, forty-four states had legislation in place that banned the substances. Florida was the second state to enact such a ban. As with Louisiana, the catalyst for the Florida ruling was a spike in bath salts–related emergencies. Specifically, a few bizarre incidents in the town of Panama City captured the attention of authorities and convinced them of how dangerous and unpredictable bath salts were.

In one case it took several police officers to subdue a man who had used his teeth to rip apart the back seat of a police car and tear out the radar unit, all the while screaming for help and saying he did not want to die. In another case a man was shooting a gun through the floor of his apartment, convinced that monsters were attacking him from below. "They're fighting things that aren't there," says Bay County sheriff Frank McKeithen. "They're hallucinating."[46] These incidents worried McKeithen so much that he shared his concerns with Florida's attorney general Pam Bondi. She agreed that they were facing a

> " A few bizarre incidents in the town of Panama City captured the attention of authorities and convinced them of how dangerous and unpredictable bath salts were. "

grave situation and that something needed to be done.

In March 2011 Bondi used the same type of emergency rule that Guidry had in Louisiana to quickly outlaw bath salts. The ban was temporary, but when it expired ninety days later, Florida's governor signed a bill that made it permanent. Since that time the state has revised its law to make it tougher, along with adding more substances to the list. State officials vow that they will continue to do this as often as necessary in order to keep synthetic drugs off the streets. Florida state senator Greg Evers explains: "We'll just do it again until we come up with the magic language."[47]

Nearly all states have also gotten aggressive about outlawing synthetic cannabinoids. In March 2010 Kansas became the first state to outlaw the use, possession, and sale of these products. Other states soon did the same, including Alabama, Georgia, Illinois, Kentucky, Michigan, Missouri, and Mississippi. By the end of November 2012 a total of forty-two states had synthetic cannabinoid laws in place.

These laws have made a positive difference, but the lack of consistency from state to state reduces their effectiveness. California's law, for instance, specifically bans certain types of synthetic marijuana, whereas other state laws focus more on the drugs' chemical compositions. Both Vermont and New Hampshire have no synthetic drug legislation, while their neighbor, Maine, has banned both synthetic cannabinoids and synthetic cathinones. Florida has outlawed an estimated ninety synthetic drugs, while New York's legislation covers only two synthetic cathinones and no cannabinoids. "The result," says the San Diego law firm Conforti and Turner, "is a Swiss-cheese-like regulatory framework that is inconsistent across state lines."[48] That situation was alleviated somewhat with legislation that was passed in July 2012. Known as the Synthetic Drug Abuse Prevention Act, this legislation has helped to solve the problem of inconsistency among states, as well as to close loopholes in the law.

## Help from the Feds

In March 2011, a year before the federal law was passed, the DEA used its emergency powers to temporarily ban five synthetic cannabinoids, including three of the most common: JWH-018, JWH-073, and JWH-200. This action made the substances illegal to manufacture, distribute, possess, import, or export. Seven months later, on October 21, 2011, the DEA took the same action with three synthetic cathinones (mephedrone, methylone, and MDPV), temporarily adding them to the Schedule I list of banned substances.

Also during 2011 the US Congress began to evaluate and debate bills that dealt with synthetic cannabinoids and cathinones. After months of debating and negotiating, the end result was the Synthetic Drug Abuse Prevention Act, which President Barack Obama signed into law on July 10, 2012. The act permanently banned fifteen synthetic cannabinoids, two synthetic cathinones, and nine 2C hallucinogens by adding them to the list of Schedule I substances. It criminalized the manufacture, distribution, use, and sale of the drugs and expanded the DEA's executive authority.

> " By the end of November 2012 a total of forty-two states had synthetic cannabinoid laws in place. "

Although the new law was hailed as the answer to an out-of-control synthetic drug epidemic, not everyone was happy with it. One critic was Glenn Duncan, executive director of the Hunterdon Drug Awareness Program in Flemington, New Jersey. Duncan, who has extensively researched synthetic drugs, criticized the Synthetic Drug Abuse Prevention Act for being a watered-down version of what was needed. Of the seventeen synthetic cathinones the DEA wanted banned as Schedule I controlled substances, only two were covered in the law. In response to reading one legislator's opinion that the law was the "final nail in the coffin for bath salts," Duncan had this to say: "It was the most ridiculous statement I ever saw. I was angered by it. If he looked at my Web site, he would see 83 substances listed. He put two nails in a coffin that needs 83 nails."[49]

## The Problem of Analogues

A major challenge faced by legislators when passing synthetic drug laws is how quickly the drugs can change. One that is banned today might become a completely different drug next week—and technically it will be legal because its name is not on a controlled substances list. This happens when chemists deliberately make changes in their drug formulas to get around the controlled substance laws, as Ryan explains: "It's like that arcade game Whac-a-Mole. Every time you think you've got a handle on it—boom—it pops up in three different places."[50]

An existing law that has been in place since 1986 was designed to address this sort of problem. The Controlled Substances Analogue Enforcement Act outlaws drug analogues, meaning substances that are chemically similar to banned drugs. The law uses three factors to define analogues: The chemical structure is close to the chemical structure of a controlled substance; the drug's effect on the central nervous system is the same or greater than the effect of a controlled substance; and the producer's intent is that the drug will have a stimulant, depressant, or hallucinogenic effect on the user.

> "A major challenge faced by legislators when passing synthetic drug laws is how quickly the drugs can change. One that is banned today might become a completely different drug next week."

In theory, the Analogue Act should criminalize and authorize prosecutions for synthetic drug analogues just like it does for analogues of drugs such as heroin or cocaine. There are challenges involved with this, however, most of which revolve around the term *human consumption*. With a controlled substance like heroin, a prosecutor can prove criminal wrongdoing simply by showing evidence that there was possession, use, and/or distribution of an illegal substance. In a court of law, there is no question what the drug's purpose was when it was made and sold. With synthetic drugs, however, devious producers intentionally mark the packages "Not for human consumption." Even though it is obvious that the phrase is being used fraudulently and the substance is indeed intended for human consumption, this is not necessarily a simple matter to prove in court. To the Maximus, a group opposed to synthetic drugs, writes:

> Greedy drug dealers have done a great job defending themselves against the Federal Analogue Act by saying that they did not intend or knowingly sell or manufacture a drug that was meant for human consumption. Ev-

eryone knows that potpourri or incense that is sold in little packages or vials by the gram is sold as a drug and not for mom to put in a bowl on the table, but this common sense is not necessarily effective in the courtroom.[51]

This issue is addressed in the Synthetic Drug Abuse Prevention Act. Not only does the law prohibit substances that are listed by name, it also outlaws "agents" produced in the future that may affect a user's brain in the same way as the original drug.

Supporters of the new federal law acknowledge that it is not perfect. Neither this nor any law is capable of removing all challenges of synthetic drug offenses, but it is considered a step in the right direction. The Maximus group writes: "Although we recognize the bill's shortcomings, it is an important start. This bill is the first federal legislation designed to begin taking a bite out of the synthetic drug industry."[52]

## The World Wide Drug Web

No matter how comprehensive and strict controlled substance laws may be, the reality is that no law can stop drug sales on the Internet. Online sales of synthetic drugs have soared in recent years, especially as regulation has made them more difficult to buy in local stores. Texas law firm Tad A. Nelson & Associates explains: "Even if bath salts and synthetic marijuana could not be sold in brick-and-mortar retail stores, they could still be easily purchased on the Internet." This problem was also addressed by the 2012 federal synthetic drug law, as the Nelson firm explains: "The federal ban applies to both interstate and online sales. Combined with existing [state] laws, the federal ban removes any question about the legality of these synthetic drugs."[53]

Yet even declaring drugs to be illegal will not stop their online dis-

> "According to DEA spokesperson Rusty Payne, the challenge of tackling illegal Internet drug sales can be overwhelming, especially when considering that thousands of websites sell the drugs."

tribution. Experts say that it is impossible for any law to completely wipe out Internet sales. Simply identifying merchants who actually operate drug websites is a daunting task, as Jeff Hahn, CEO of the Minneapolis firm Internet Exposure explains: "Anyone who wants to cover up their involvement in a website can register a domain with false information or use a domain privacy service."[54] Such privacy services exist for the sole purpose of concealing the identities of their clients, and many are very good at what they do.

According to DEA spokesperson Rusty Payne, the challenge of tackling illegal Internet drug sales can be overwhelming, especially when considering that thousands of websites sell the drugs. "Unfortunately," he says, "there are underground labs all over the world who ship their products globally to customers. DEA works with other countries to attack these global drug networks, but we do not have the legal authority to shut a website down immediately when discovered."[55] In cases where the agency has managed to shut down a synthetic drug site, officials have been frustrated by how quickly the site operators were able to get up and running again at a different location on the Internet.

## No Simple Answers

Health officials, state legislators, and members of Congress have all done their part to address the synthetic drug problem. Numerous laws have been passed and were specifically written so they can be revised as necessary. Regulating synthetic drugs is a significant challenge, however, and there is every indication that it will remain so in the foreseeable future. "This stuff is not going away," says Payne. "We are going to be dealing with synthetic use for a long time."[56]

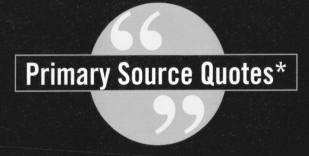

# How Should Synthetic Drugs Be Regulated?

66 **Criminalizing these drugs at the federal level would result in interfering with states' ability to control their own drug policies.** 99

—Rand Paul, letter to US senators Amy Klobuchar and Charles Grassley, December 14, 2011.
http://blogs.courier-journal.com.

Paul is a US senator from Kentucky.

66 **The problem with relying on state bans is that what is banned in one state is legal in another. We need to pass our bill for a federal ban on synthetic marijuana. . . . All we need is one senator, Rand Paul of Kentucky, to release his block on this legislation.** 99

—Charles Schumer, "We Need National Legislation to Ban 'Synthetic Pot,'" *New York Daily News*, March 21, 2012.
www.nydailynews.com.

Schumer is a US senator from New York.

Bracketed quotes indicate conflicting positions.

* Editor's Note: While the definition of a primary source can be narrowly or broadly defined, for the purposes of Compact Research, a primary source consists of: 1) results of original research presented by an organization or researcher; 2) eyewitness accounts of events, personal experience, or work experience; 3) first-person editorials offering pundits' opinions; 4) government officials presenting political plans and/or policies; 5) representatives of organizations presenting testimony or policy.

Primary Source Quotes

66 Every time one chemical gets banned, makers substitute another chemical, chemically virtually identical in its composition and effects, to circumvent a ban. The solution to implement a broader, widespread ban on synthetic chemicals has yet to overcome legislative hurdles. 99

—Gregory Bunt, "Synthetic Marijuana: A New Clear and Present Danger," *Huffington Post*, February 22, 2012. www.huffingtonpost.com.

Bunt is medical director and senior vice president of Health Services at the New York residential treatment facility Daytop Village.

66 The U.S. Drug Enforcement Administration has made the possession of the chemicals used to make bath salts illegal, but that hasn't stopped people from making and using the substances. 99

—Margaret Larson, "Recognizing Signs of Bath Salts," Global Good Group, August 28, 2012. http://globalgoodgroup.com.

Larson is a nurse and public health educator from Texas.

66 Placing synthetic cannabinoid and synthetic stimulant substances in schedule I would expose those who manufacture, distribute, possess, import, and export synthetic drugs without proper authority to the full spectrum of criminal, civil, and administrative penalties, sanctions, and regulatory controls. 99

—Ronald Weich, letter to the Honorable F. James Sensenbrenner Jr., September 30, 2011. www.justice.gov.

Weich is the assistant US attorney general.

❝While it is too soon to discern the overall public health impact of the abuse of synthetic cannabinoids, previous experience with other designer drugs shows that making synthetic drugs illegal does not prevent them from being made and abused.❞

—Jenny L. Wiley, Julie A. Marusich, John W. Huffman, Robert L. Balster, and Brian F. Thomas, "Hijacking of Basic Research: The Case of Synthetic Cannabinoids," RTI International, November 2011. www.rti.org.

Wiley, Marusich, and Thomas are researchers with RTI International, Balster is director of the Institute for Drug and Alcohol Studies, and Huffman is a retired organic chemist who first created synthetic cannabinoids.

❝'Bath Salts' and the like have never been regulated by the Food and Drug Administration (FDA) because the components were not recognized as food or drugs.❞

—Bonnie Nolan, "Are 'Bath Salts' Just Hype?," *Psychology Today*, October 3, 2012. www.psychologytoday.com.

Nolan is a neuroscientist and lecturer at Rutgers University.

❝Designer drugs have been synthesized and marketed for decades, with or without controlled substance laws. Wherever there is a niche market, someone, somewhere will try to permeate it for profit.❞

—Bertha K. Madras, "Designer Drugs: An Escalating Public Health Challenge," *Journal of Global Drug Policy and Practice*, September 10, 2012. www.globaldrugpolicy.org.

Madras is a professor in the Department of Psychiatry at Harvard Medical School.

❝Despite federal and state regulations to prohibit [synthetic cannabinoid] sale and distribution, illicit use continues, and reports of illness are increasing.❞

—Tracy D. Murphy et al., "Acute Kidney Injury Associated with Synthetic Cannabinoid Use—Multiple States, 2012," *Morbidity and Mortality Weekly Report*, Centers for Disease Control and Prevention, February 15, 2013. www.cdc.gov.

Murphy is a clinical pathologist from Cheyenne, Wyoming.

# Facts and Illustrations

## How Should Synthetic Drugs Be Regulated?

- In October 2011 bath salts were put on **Schedule I** of the Controlled Substances Act, which indicated that the drugs have no legitimate use or safety in the United States and are highly addictive.

- According to February 28, 2013, data from the American Association of Poison Control Centers, the number of bath salts–related calls to US poison centers dropped from 6,136 in 2011 to 2,655 in 2012; health officials believe this is at least partly due to **tougher regulations** on synthetic drugs that were passed in 2011 and 2012.

- In 2009 the United Kingdom amended the Drugs Act of 1971 to list synthetic cannabinoids as controlled substances; rather than deterring the sale and use of synthetic drugs, the ban **spurred development** of new synthetic cannabinoid products.

- Although certain synthetic cannabinoids and/or specific chemicals contained in these preparations were made illegal in some states, a **comprehensive national ban** was not enacted until July 2012.

- According to the Substance Abuse and Mental Health Services Administration, the Synthetic Drug Abuse Prevention Act of 2012 prohibits not only currently identified **chemical cocktails** used in bath salts and synthetic marijuana but all **similar compounds** that might be produced in the future.

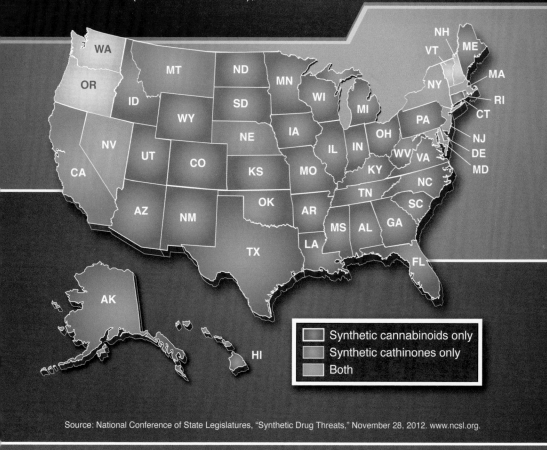

## Most States Have Banned Synthetic Drugs

Nearly all US states have joined the federal government in passing laws that regulate synthetic drugs. This map shows those states that have banned synthetic cannabinoids (used in Spice or K2), synthetic cathinones (used in bath salts), or both.

Synthetic cannabinoids only
Synthetic cathinones only
Both

Source: National Conference of State Legislatures, "Synthetic Drug Threats," November 28, 2012. www.ncsl.org.

- According to the White House Office of National Drug Control Policy, prior to 2010 synthetic cannabinoids were not controlled by any **state or federal law**.

- According to a report by the National Conference of State Legislatures, as of November 28, 2012, at least **forty-five states** and Puerto Rico had banned synthetic cannabinoids and/or bath salts.

# Federal Efforts to Stop Synthetic Drug Abuse

In an attempt to gain control of the rapidly growing problem of synthetic drug abuse in the United States, the federal government implemented temporary bans in 2011 and a permanent ban in 2012. This diagram shows the various legislative actions that were taken.

| Date | Action |
|------|--------|
| **March 2011** | Five synthetic cannabinoids (used to make synthetic marijuana) were temporarily categorized by the Drug Enforcement Administration (DEA) as Schedule I controlled substances. |
| **October 2011** | The DEA exercised its emergency scheduling authority to categorize three synthetic cathinones (used to make bath salts) as Schedule I substances. |
| **December 2011** | The US House of Representatives approved legislation that bans certain synthetic drugs. |
| **July 2012** | The US Congress passed the Synthetic Drug Abuse Prevention Act, and President Barack Obama signed it into law. |

Source: Substance Abuse and Mental Health Services Administration, "Will They Turn You into a Zombie? What Clinicians Need to Know About Synthetic Drugs: Trainer Guide," September 25, 2012. www.uclaisap.org.

- The Synthetic Drug Abuse Prevention Act of 2012 outlaws both **interstate and Internet sales** of chemical cocktails used to make bath salts and synthetic marijuana.

- In January 2011 Louisiana became the first US state to pass legislation that **banned six synthetic cathinones** found in bath salts.

- When the Drug Enforcement Administration designated certain synthetic drugs as Schedule I controlled substances, this put the drugs in the same category as **LSD, heroin, and marijuana**.

## Steady Decline in Bath Salts Use Post-Regulation

After a massive spike in bath salts–related emergencies between 2010 and 2011, calls to poison control centers nationwide continued to inch upward during the first months of 2012. Then in mid-year the calls began to taper off, and by December the number had dropped to 81 compared with 422 the previous June. Although health officials cannot be certain what caused the decline, they say it could be related to tougher federal legislation passed in July 2012, combined with more stringent state laws.

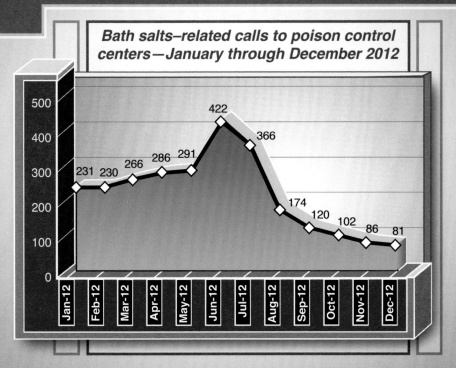

**Bath salts–related calls to poison control centers—January through December 2012**

Source: American Association of Poison Control Centers, "Bath Salts Data," March 31, 2013. http://aapcc.s3.amazonaws.com.

- After the Synthetic Drug Abuse Prevention Act became law in July 2012, bath salts–related calls to poison control centers dropped to **81** by the end of the year, from a high of **422** in June.

- In October 2011 the Council of the European Union adopted a pact against synthetic drugs to help countries more effectively **control production and trafficking** of the drugs.

# How Can Synthetic Drug Abuse Be Prevented?

> **Research shows that preventing drug use before it begins is a cost-effective, common-sense approach to promoting safe and healthy communities.**
>
> —R. Gil Kerlikowske, director of the Office of National Drug Control Policy.

> **This synthetic drug problem is bad, it's getting worse, it's affecting our youth—killing many of them. We need to continue educating our children as to the severe dangers of these poisonous chemicals.**
>
> —David Seaberg, president of the American College of Emergency Physicians.

Mike and Jan Rozga continue to mourn the death of their eighteen-year-old son David, and their grief may never fade away. But as difficult as it is to talk about the tragedy, they believe the best way to honor David's memory is by sharing his story with teens. By doing so, they might be able to save other young people from his fate—being driven to suicide after smoking synthetic marijuana. In April 2011 testimony at a US Senate hearing, Mike Rozga stated: "David was mentally and physically attacked by the K2, causing hallucinations, unimaginable anxiety, and loss of his ability to reason. If he and his friends had known then what we know now, they never would have smoked the stuff. We are firmly convinced that David would still be alive today had he not smoked K2."[57]

## Vowing to Make a Difference

At the time of his death, David had just graduated from high school in Indianola, Iowa, and was making plans to start college in the fall. While he was spending some time celebrating graduation with his friends, someone brought out a packet of K2 that was purchased legally at a local store. Even though a couple of people tried to talk him out of it, David decided to smoke the drug—and less than two hours later was dead of a self-inflicted gunshot wound. His parents and younger brother Daniel were shattered. They knew that David was not the type of person to take his own life. He was healthy, happy, athletic, popular, and had a bright future ahead. On a website dedicated to him, the Rozgas write: "Unaware of his K2 use, we began to do what any family would do. Immediately and desperately, we searched for an explanation. Why? Why would David take his own life? What warning signs did we miss? Questions spiraled, but answers could not be found."[58]

Two days after David's death, his family found out about the drug he had taken and the horrible effects it had on him. "We know now," says Mike Rozga, "that David was tortured both mentally and physically before he died. This drug puts you in a place where you will do anything to escape it and reality means nothing."[59] The Rozgas' anger over the senselessness of their son's death fueled their passion to share their message with young people. They gave their first talk about what happened to David—and the dangers of synthetic marijuana—at his funeral in front of more than a thousand people. Even in the midst of unbearable grief, they felt the need to do something to get the message out.

> Educating teens about the dangers of synthetic drugs is becoming a priority of schools and community organizations throughout the United States.

In the years since David's death the Rozgas have done numerous local and national interviews on the radio and on television, made public service announcements, and delivered presentations at schools, colleges, churches, and clubs. The family also founded a drug prevention organization called Standing Together On Prevention (STOP) and created a website called K2 Drug Facts.

In October 2012 Mike, Jan, and Daniel Rozga received a prestigious award from the White House for their work to help prevent synthetic drug use among young people. The Advocates for Action award is given each year to select Americans who have worked hard to help improve the health and safety of their communities. The Rozgas say they were humbled by the honor and plan to continue the work they have started: Says Mike Rozga:

> At the time our son David died in June 2010 after smoking K2, virtually no one had heard of this synthetic drug. There was literally no information from the scientific community available—it was just too new. We made a decision very early on that we needed to do something; we needed to share our story in the hope that we could prevent this from happening to another family. . . . This has been a slow, difficult, and painful process, but we know we are making a difference.[60]

## Cooperative Efforts

Educating teens about the dangers of synthetic drugs is becoming a priority of schools and community organizations throughout the United States. In Johnson City, Tennessee, for instance, the sheriff's department has joined forces with the county school system to help spread awareness about synthetic drugs and educate the public about them. Sheriff Ed Graybeal is convinced that the first line of defense against substance abuse begins in the classroom. "The more education we put out there," says Graybeal, "the more power these students are going to have to make the right decision when they come across this stuff."[61] The program involves members of law enforcement going into schools to teach students about the health effects and risks of synthetic drugs. The group also hosts forums for parents and community members.

The reaction of teens who have attended presentations has been positive. They have expressed that they gained knowledge they did not have before, such as learning about the harmful effects that often result from taking a synthetic drug. They have also learned that taking the drugs has consequences that they may not have considered before the presentation. Some, like high school student Aaron Ford, remarked afterward that what they learned strengthened their resolve to stay away from synthetic drugs. "They clarified that it wasn't really a scare tactic," says Ford, "where the drugs themselves are so scary, just knowing the facts, it definitely scared a lot of people. It scared me off from even thinking about it."[62]

> "Deceptive Danger videos tell real-life stories of people from Tennessee who have been struggling with addictions to either prescription medicines or synthetic drugs.

Another area of the country where law enforcement professionals are partnering with schools is Clarkston, Michigan. During an October 2012 forum at a middle school, presenters included a district court judge, deputies from the county sheriff's office, and experts in drug and behavioral counseling. A young man attended as a guest of the judge: twenty-year-old Jeremy Byers, who had previously been in trouble with the law for possession and abuse of synthetic marijuana. Byers spoke to parents and teens in the audience about his history with the drug, the bad choices he made along the way, and how terrible a substance it is. "This should be illegal," Byers said. "It's one of the top-worst drugs out there."[63]

## Deceptive Danger

In October 2012 a synthetic and prescription drug abuse prevention program was launched in Tennessee. Its name, Deceptive Danger, evolved from the realization that young people are often deceived into thinking that all substances are safe as long as they are prescribed by doctors or purchased over the counter at a convenience store—neither of which is true. The program was organized in 2012 by the Tennessee District Attorneys General Conference. It includes an educational Deceptive Danger DVD, posters that focus on either prescription drugs or synthetic drugs, and a brochure that covers both types of drug abuse and the legal consequences. Another important element of the program is presentations that district attorneys give at high schools throughout the state.

The Deceptive Danger videos tell real-life stories of people from Tennessee who have been struggling with addictions to either prescription medicines or synthetic drugs. Guy Jones, deputy director of the Tennessee District Attorneys General Conference, shares his thoughts about the value of the program: "Prescription medication and synthetic drug abuse is a growing problem in Tennessee, and one that we must curb as quickly as possible. The Deceptive Danger campaign gives our DAs a chance to show young Tennesseans the repercussions of using these drugs that may appear relatively harmless to them at first. Everyone needs to know these drugs are very dangerous."[64]

## Committed Media

For the editorial staff at the Minneapolis, Minnesota, newspaper *Star Tribune*, the focus on synthetic drugs began with a story in March 2011; specifically, the tragic account of the drug-related death of Trevor Robinson after the party in Blaine. "Ever since that day last spring," says editor Nancy Barnes, "when a group of Minnesota teenagers and young adults overdosed on a synthetic substance none of us had ever heard of, this news organization has focused on understanding a new wave of drugs with the hopes of preventing other overdoses and deaths." Barnes goes on to say that the journalists who worked on the story gained a wealth of knowledge about how "deceptively dangerous these synthetic drugs are, why they are so readily available, who is profiting from their sale, and how difficult it is to crack down on dealers."[65]

> "Staff at the newspaper agreed that the knowledge was too valuable not to share, so they used it to develop an educational program."

Staff at the newspaper agreed that the knowledge was too valuable not to share, so they used it to develop an educational program. Barnes writes: "We've come to the sobering realization that neither local nor national law enforcement officials will be able to keep this problem in check without broad and sustained educational efforts."[66] Newspaper staff created educational videos with excerpts from some of the news reports and made educational DVDs available to schools throughout Minnesota.

One of the videos features firsthand accounts from four of the teens who were at the Blaine party, including Jesse Fisher, A.J. Carver, and two others. Says Barnes: "These young people decided to publicly share their memories of what happened that night in March 2011, and what they learned from the experience, with the hope that others would learn from this tragic event."[67] A second video features interviews with Dan Moren, the DEA's top representative in Minnesota, and Cody Wiberg, who is executive director of the Minnesota Board of Pharmacy. The two describe the growing problems caused by synthetic drugs, explain what the substances are, and discuss how they affect the body.

To raise awareness of the prevention program, the *Star Tribune* worked with the Minnesota School Counselors Association, which e-mailed nearly eight hundred members and invited them to request the video. "Within minutes of delivery," says Barnes, "we started hearing back from school counselors, with one asking for as many as 10 copies of the DVD. At the same time, the counselors wrote us about their own struggles with synthetic-drug use at their schools." Barnes is very enthusiastic about the program. She is also grateful to everyone who helped make it a reality—especially the teens from Blaine who agreed to participate even in the midst of grieving the death of their friend. "We'd like to say thank you to the young adults who worked with us on this project." says Barnes. "Hopefully, their willingness to speak out will help save a life."[68]

> " As awareness continues to grow about the dangers of bath salts, synthetic marijuana, and synthetic hallucinogens such as 2C-E, the number of educational prevention programs will undoubtedly grow too. "

## Lives at Stake

Law enforcement professionals, health officials, educators, legislators, and addiction experts agree that synthetic drugs represent a daunting challenge. As with any type of substance abuse or addiction, preventing the problem before it occurs is always better than attempting to fix it afterward. Because synthetic drugs have not been around very long, education and awareness programs are much scarcer than they are for alcohol, marijuana, or other illicit drugs, but that is starting to change.

As awareness continues to grow about the dangers of bath salts, synthetic marijuana, and synthetic hallucinogens such as 2C-E, the number of educational prevention programs will undoubtedly grow too. For families such as the Rogzas, who have suffered a terrible loss, the growth of these programs will not bring back their loved ones. It may, however, bring them some comfort knowing that some good resulted from tragedy. They write: "We pray that David's legacy will be found in the way he enjoyed life and, most importantly, in the lives that might be saved because of his story."[69]

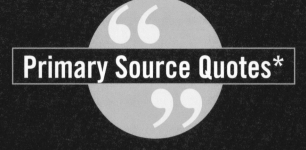

## Primary Source Quotes*

# How Can Synthetic Drug Abuse Be Prevented?

66 When discussing drugs of abuse with my students, I often ask what, if anything, convinces students themselves to avoid drugs. The overwhelming response is that they respond to facts, rather than hype. 99

—Bonnie Nolan, "Are 'Bath Salts' Just Hype?," *Psychology Today*, October 3, 2012. www.psychologytoday.com.

Nolan is a neuroscientist and lecturer at Rutgers University.

66 Healthcare professionals, law enforcement, testing capabilities, a massive public education campaign and strategies for deterrence in healthcare systems are needed to respond to this emerging threat. 99

—Bertha K. Madras, "Designer Drugs: An Escalating Public Health Challenge," *Journal of Global Drug Policy and Practice*, September 10, 2012. www.globaldrugpolicy.org.

Madras is a professor in the Department of Psychiatry at Harvard Medical School.

* Editor's Note: While the definition of a primary source can be narrowly or broadly defined, for the purposes of Compact Research, a primary source consists of: 1) results of original research presented by an organization or researcher; 2) eyewitness accounts of events, personal experience, or work experience; 3) first-person editorials offering pundits' opinions; 4) government officials presenting political plans and/or policies; 5) representatives of organizations presenting testimony or policy.

Primary Source Quotes

**66** One of the most important elements of primary prevention is education—providing credible, easy-to-understand information on the harmful consequences of psychoactive substance use. **99**

—Darryl S. Inaba and William E. Cohen, *Uppers, Downers, All Arounders*. Medford, OR: CNS Productions, 2011, p. 12.

Inaba is a pharmacist and expert on drugs and addiction, and Cohen is an educator and filmmaker.

**66** Educating children and young people about the risks of synthetic drugs is crucial. **99**

—*Rapid City (SD) Journal*, "Editorial: Synthetic Drugs Should Be Illegal," February 5, 2012. http://rapidcityjournal.com.

The *Rapid City (SD) Journal* is the daily newspaper of Rapid City, South Dakota, and the second largest newspaper in the state.

**66** Raising awareness and educating the public is crucial in putting a stop to the synthetic drug epidemic. **99**

—Council on Chemical Abuse, "Synthetic Drugs: Unstable & Dangerous," Fact Sheet, February 2, 2012. www.councilonchemicalabuse.org.

Located in Reading, Pennsylvania, the Council on Chemical Abuse serves as the coordinating agency for publicly supported programming on drug and alcohol abuse throughout the county.

**66** To a considerable degree, prevention must occur drug by drug, because people will not necessarily generalize the adverse consequences of one drug to the use of others. **99**

—Lloyd D. Johnston, Patrick M. O'Malley, Jerald G. Bachman, and John E. Schulenberg, *Monitoring the Future: National Results on Drug Use*, February 2013. www.monitoringthefuture.org.

Johnston, O'Malley, Bachman, and Schulenberg are researchers with the University of Michigan Institute for Social Research.

**❝Educators can help prevent use of synthetic canna-binoids by addressing use of these substances in pro-grams designed to prevent use of illicit drugs.❞**

—Substance Abuse and Mental Health Services Administration, "Drug-Related Emergency Department Visits Involving Synthetic Cannabinoids," *DAWN Report*, December 4, 2012. www.samhsa.gov.

The SAMHSA seeks to reduce the impact of substance abuse and mental illness on America's communities.

·····································································································································································

**❝Gateway Foundation believes that communicating the dangerous and damaging effects of synthetic drugs like K2 and bath salts abuse through public awareness and education is critical.❞**

—Gateway Foundation, "K2 & Bath Salts: Understanding Synthetic Drugs," August 2012. http://recovergateway.org.

Gateway Foundation is the largest provider of substance abuse treatment in the state of Illinois.

·····································································································································································

## How Can Synthetic Drug Abuse Be Prevented?

- In a December 2012 report the Substance Abuse and Mental Health Services Administration states that parents can help prevent their children from obtaining synthetic drugs by setting **parental controls for all online purchases**.

- The National Institute on Drug Abuse states that teenagers respond more to **science-based facts** about how synthetic drugs affect the body than to scare tactics.

- In an effort to prevent people's ability to obtain synthetic drugs, Japan has banned fifty-four compounds that are known as **precursors**, meaning substances used to make the drugs.

- In March 2013 fifty-five countries voted to create an **early warning system**, which will enable more advanced countries to share data more quickly with less advanced nations when investigators first hear of new synthetic compounds.

- According to Ohio drug abuse prevention specialist Jim Ryan, substance abuse among teens is not likely to begin with synthetic drugs but with alcohol or natural marijuana; thus, a strong stance against underage drinking and smoking pot is a crucial first step for any **prevention program**.

## Teens Lack Awareness of Synthetic Drug Risks

Young people who are unaware of the risks of synthetic drugs are more likely to use them. And, according to the 2012 *Monitoring the Future* survey of eighth, tenth, and twelfth graders, most do not perceive the use of these drugs as risky. These findings demonstrate the need for strong prevention efforts, especially education.

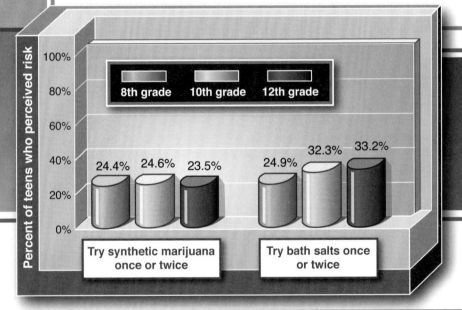

**How much do you think people risk harming themselves (physically or in other ways) if they . . .**

Percent of teens who perceived risk

- 8th grade
- 10th grade
- 12th grade

Try synthetic marijuana once or twice: 24.4%, 24.6%, 23.5%

Try bath salts once or twice: 24.9%, 32.3%, 33.2%

Source: Lloyd D. Johnston, Patrick M. O'Malley, Jerald G. Bachman, and John E. Schulenberg, *Monitoring the Future: National Results on Drug Use*, February 2013. www.monitoringthefuture.org.

- According to the National Institute on Drug Abuse, drug prevention programs should be long-term with **repeated interventions** (such as "booster programs") to reinforce the original prevention goals. This is because studies have shown that the benefits from middle school prevention programs diminish without follow-up programs in high school.

# Nearly $1.4 Billion Spent on Substance Abuse Prevention

US government statistics from 2012 show that 22.6 million Americans over the age of twelve were illicit drug users during 2010, which was the highest overall rate since 2002. Because widespread illicit drug abuse results in significant social, public health, and economic problems, federal government agencies allocate tens of millions of dollars each year for prevention and treatment programs. During 2012, these collectively totaled $1.4 billion. Shown on this chart are the various agencies and their allocations toward substance abuse prevention in the United States.

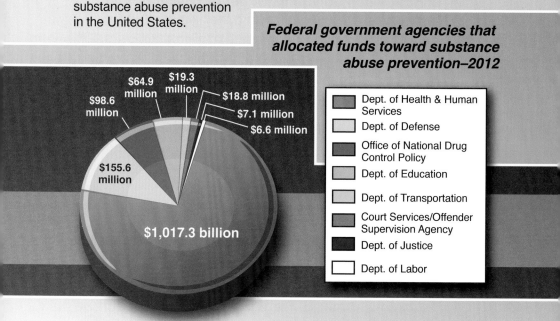

**Federal government agencies that allocated funds toward substance abuse prevention–2012**

$64.9 million
$19.3 million
$98.6 million
$18.8 million
$7.1 million
$6.6 million
$155.6 million
$1,017.3 billion

- Dept. of Health & Human Services
- Dept. of Defense
- Office of National Drug Control Policy
- Dept. of Education
- Dept. of Transportation
- Court Services/Offender Supervision Agency
- Dept. of Justice
- Dept. of Labor

Source: US Government Accountability Office, "Initial Review of the National Strategy and Drug Abuse Prevention and Treatment Programs," July 6, 2012. www.gao.gov.

- A July 2012 sting operation called Operation Log Jam resulted in an enormous amount of synthetic drug seizures, including **4.8 million** packets of synthetic cannabinoids and products to make **13 million** more packets, as well as 167,000 packets of synthetic cathinones and the products to make an additional 392,000 packets.

- In March 2013 the US Navy launched an education and awareness campaign with the focus on preventing the use of synthetic drugs while emphasizing the importance of **bystander involvement and intervention**.

- According to Ohio drug abuse prevention specialist Jim Ryan, **social workers** play a key role in synthetic drug use prevention and awareness efforts.

- Child and adolescent psychiatrist Joseph Lee emphasizes that it is a risky mistake to wait for young people to show signs of addiction before educating them about synthetic drugs; rather, **preventive measures** should be in place long before danger signs appear.

- According to the National Institute on Drug Abuse, drug prevention programs are most effective when they employ interactive techniques, such as **peer discussion groups and parent role-playing**, that allow for active involvement in learning about drug abuse and reinforcing skills.

# Key People and Advocacy Groups

**Lazăr Edeleanu:** A Romanian chemist who in 1887 was the first person to synthesize amphetamine.

**Richard A. Glennon:** A medicinal chemist who was the first to develop a synthetic cathinone, the psychoactive ingredient found in the shrub *Catha edulis* (khat).

**Allyn Howlett:** An American scientist who was the first to prove that humans have cannabinoid receptors in the brain.

**John W. Huffman:** A chemist who was the first to synthesize cannabinoids in his laboratory at Clemson University in South Carolina.

**National Institute on Drug Abuse (NIDA):** An agency of the National Institutes of Health, the NIDA seeks to end drug abuse and addiction in the United States.

**Office of National Drug Control Policy:** A component of the Executive Office of the President, this agency is responsible for directing the federal government's antidrug programs.

**Partnership at Drugfree.org:** An organization that is committed to helping parents and families solve the problem of teenage substance abuse.

**Mark Ryan:** A physician who directs the Louisiana Poison Control Center, Ryan was among the first to document the significant rise in bath salts abuse and to alert health officials about it.

**Alexander Shulgin:** A California pharmacologist who, with permission of the US Drug Enforcement Administration, developed the 2C family of synthetic hallucinogenic drugs and tested many of them on himself. These were to be used only for research, and when Shulgin became an admitted enthusiast of his creations, the DEA pulled his license.

**US Drug Enforcement Administration (DEA):** The lead agency for domestic enforcement of federal drug laws as well as for coordinating and pursuing US drug investigations abroad.

**Nora Volkow:** The director of the National Institute on Drug Abuse (NIDA), who often speaks to groups about the dangers of substance abuse among youth and the growing problem with synthetic drugs.

# Chronology

**1928**
The first synthetic cathinone is produced by Russian scientists and is used as an antidepressant; decades pass before researchers outside the Soviet Union learn of the discovery.

**1929**
The chemical mephedrone is first described by pharmacologist Saem de Burnaga Sanchez in an article that appears in a French scientific journal.

**1987**
Medicinal chemist Richard A. Glennon publishes a paper in the journal *Pharmacology, Biochemistry and Behavior*, in which he describes his creation of a synthetic cathinone.

**1982**
After injecting contaminated synthetic heroin, a group of addicts in Northern California develops a severe, permanent nerve disorder that is nearly identical to advanced Parkinson's disease. It later becomes known as the United States's first "designer drug disaster."

**1930**   **1960**   **1975**   **1990**

**1964**
Israeli chemist Raphael Mechoulam is the first to isolate the psychoactive substance tetrahydrocannabinol (THC) from the *Cannabis sativa* plant.

**1970**
Congress passes the Comprehensive Drug Abuse Prevention and Control Act (Controlled Substances Act), which establishes five "schedules" for the classification and control of drug substances that are subject to abuse.

**1984**
The Comprehensive Crime Control Act amends the Controlled Substances Act to authorize the US attorney general to temporarily ban substances that pose an "imminent hazard to the public safety."

**1986**
Congress passes the Controlled Substances Analogue Enforcement Act, which makes it illegal to distribute drugs that are chemically similar to (analogues of) existing Schedule I substances.

**1988**
American scientist Allyn Howlett proves that humans have cannabinoid receptors in the brain.

**1991**

California pharmacologist Alexander Shulgin publishes a book called *PiHKAL: A Chemical Love Story* in which he reveals his formulas for the 2C family of hallucinogenic synthetic drugs.

**2011**

The US Drug Enforcement Administration orders a temporary ban on five synthetic cannabinoids; later the same year the agency also bans three synthetic cathinones.

**2010**

Kansas becomes the first state to outlaw the use, possession, and sale of synthetic cannabinoids; later the same year Louisiana becomes the first state to ban synthetic cathinones.

**1995**

Clemson University organic chemistry professor John W. Huffman creates a synthetic cannabinoid compound known as JWH-018.

**2009**

At least twenty-one countries in the European Union report the presence of synthetic marijuana.

**1990**

**2000**

**2010**

**1993**

Natural cathinone (from the khat plant) is banned by the US Drug Enforcement Administration as a Schedule I substance, meaning it has a high potential for abuse and no recognized medicinal value.

**2007**

In the first known appearance of MDPV (the powerful stimulant used in bath salts), a sample of the substance is seized by law enforcement officials in Germany.

**2008**

The first shipment of Spice (synthetic marijuana) is seized and analyzed by US Customs and Border Patrol in Dayton, Ohio.

**2012**

President Barack Obama signs the Synthetic Drug Abuse Prevention Act into law, which permanently bans twenty-six synthetic drugs by classifying them as Schedule I controlled substances.

**2013**

Legislation that would criminalize the synthetic hallucinogen 25-I, along with more than two dozen other synthetic drugs, is passed by the Criminal Justice Committee of the US House of Representatives.

# Related Organizations

## American Association of Poison Control Centers (AAPCC)

515 King St., Suite 510
Alexandria, VA 22314
phone: (703) 894-1858
e-mail: info@aapcc.org • website: www.aapcc.org

The AAPCC is the parent organization for fifty-seven poison control centers throughout the United States and maintains the country's only comprehensive poisoning surveillance database. Its website offers a large collection of data and statistics about synthetic drugs.

## Council on Chemical Abuse

601 Penn St., Suite 600
Reading, PA 19601
phone: (610) 376-8669 • fax: (610) 376-8423
website: www.councilonchemicalabuse.org

The Council on Chemical Abuse serves as the coordinating agency for publicly supported programming on drug and alcohol abuse throughout Berks County. A number of articles and fact sheets about synthetic drugs are available through its website.

## Drug Free America Foundation

5999 Central Ave., Suite 301
Saint Petersburg, FL 33710
phone: (727) 828-0211 • fax: (727) 828-0212
e-mail: webmaster@dfaf.org • website: www.dfaf.org

The Drug Free America Foundation is a drug prevention and policy organization. Its website has a search engine that produces numerous articles about bath salts and other synthetic drugs, and it also has links to a site for young people titled Students Taking Action Not Drugs (STAND).

## Drug Policy Alliance

131 West 33rd St., 15th Floor
New York, NY 10001
phone: (212) 613-8020 • fax: (212) 613-8021
e-mail: nyc@drugpolicy.org • website: www.drugpolicy.org

The Drug Policy Alliance promotes alternatives to current drug policy that are grounded in science, compassion, health, and human rights. Its website features drug facts, statistics, information about drug laws, and a search engine that produces a number of articles about synthetic drugs.

## National Institute on Drug Abuse (NIDA)

National Institutes of Health
6001 Executive Blvd., Room 5213
Bethesda, MD 20892
phone: (301) 443-1124
e-mail: information@nida.nih.gov • website: www.drugabuse.gov

The NIDA supports research efforts and ensures the rapid dissemination of research to improve drug abuse prevention, treatment, and policy. The website links to a separate "NIDA for Teens" site, which is designed especially for teenagers and provides a wealth of information about drugs, including bath salts and other synthetic drugs.

## Office of National Drug Control Policy

750 Seventeenth St. NW
Washington, DC 20503
phone: (800) 666-3332 • fax: (202) 395–6708
e-mail: ondcp@ncjrs.org • website: www.whitehouse.gov/ondcp

A component of the Executive Office of the President, the Office of National Drug Control Policy is responsible for directing the federal government's antidrug programs. A wide variety of publications about bath salts and other synthetic drugs can be accessed through the site's search engine.

## Partnership at Drugfree.org

352 Park Ave. South, 9th Floor
New York, NY 10010
phone: (212) 922-1560 • fax: (212) 922-1570
website: www.drugfree.org

The Partnership at Drugfree.org is dedicated to helping parents and families solve the problem of teenage substance abuse. Its website offers a large variety of informative publications that can be accessed through the search engine, including many on bath salts and other synthetic drugs.

## Substance Abuse and Mental Health Services Administration (SAMHSA)

1 Choke Cherry Rd.
Rockville, MD 20857
phone: (877) 726-4727 • fax: (240) 221-4292
e-mail: SAMHSAInfo@samhsa.hhs.gov • website: www.samhsa.gov

The SAMHSA's mission is to reduce the impact of substance abuse and mental illness on America's communities. The site offers a wealth of information about substance abuse, and numerous publications related to bath salts and other synthetic drugs can be produced through its search engine.

## To the Maximus Foundation

1120 Grenada Dr.
Aurora, IL 60506
phone: (630) 892-3629
e-mail: info@2themax.org • website: http://2themax.org

Created in memory of a young man who died after using synthetic marijuana, To the Maximus Foundation is committed to education about and awareness of the dangers of synthetic drugs. Its website offers news releases, fact sheets, testimonials, and links to other resources and a blog.

## US Drug Enforcement Administration (DEA)

2401 Jefferson Davis Hwy.
Alexandria, VA 22301
phone: (202) 307-1000; toll-free: (800) 332-4288
website: www.justice.gov/dea

The DEA is the United States' top federal drug law enforcement agency. Its website links to a separate site called "Just Think Twice" that is designed for teenagers and offers fact sheets, personal experiences, and a search engine that produces numerous publications about bath salts and other synthetic drugs.

# For Further Research

## Books

Raymond Goldberg, *Drugs Across the Spectrum*. Belmont, CA: Wadsworth, 2012.

Howard Samuels with Jane O'Boyle, *Alive Again: Recovering from Alcoholism and Drug Addiction*. Hoboken, NJ: John Wiley & Sons, 2013.

Russ Taylor, *Bath Salts*. CreateSpace, 2012.

## Periodicals

Amos Barshad and Annie Ferrer, "Salts Tripping: The Latest Very-Bad-for-You Designer Drug Has Nothing to Do with the Stuff That Goes in a Tub," *New York*, February 21, 2011.

John DiConsiglio, "This Drug Shouldn't Be Out There," *Scholastic Choices*, February/March 2011.

David DiSalvo, "'Bath Salts' Are Evolving and Law Makers Can't Keep Up," *Forbes*, July 28, 2012.

*Economist*, "The Synthetic Scare: Bath Salts," August 4, 2012.

Anita Hassan, "Dangerous Designer Drug Hits the Streets," *Houston Chronicle*, September 23, 2012.

Pam Louwagie, "Blaine Party Survivors: 'All of Us Could Have Died That Night,'" *Minneapolis Star Tribune*, December 19, 2011.

Ashley Mateo, "I Over Dosed on Synthetic Drugs!," *Seventeen*, June/July 2012.

Larry Oakes, "Synthetic Drug Sales Booming on Web," *Minneapolis Star Tribune*, September 11, 2011.

Mehmet Oz, "'Bath Salts': Evil Lurking at Your Corner Store," *Time*, April 25, 2011.

Erinn Singman-Kaine, "Emerging Drugs: Building Awareness Within Formations," *Military Police*, Fall 2011.

Mikelle D. Smith, "Spice: A Temporary High for a Permanent Change," *All Hands*, September 2011.

Jacob Sullivan, "Bath Salts Face Off: Synthetic Drug Ban," *Reason*, October 2012.

Jennifer Van Pelt, "Synthetic Drugs—Fake Substances, Real Dangers," *Social Work Today*, July/August 2012.

## Internet Sources

Glenn Duncan, "Comprehensive Drug Information on Synthetic Cannabinoids—'Spice' and 'K2,'" Hunterdon Drug Awareness Program, June 29, 2012. www.hdap.org/spice.html.

Dirk Hanson, "The Year in Synthetic Drugs," *Salon*, December 26, 2012. www.salon.com/2012/12/26/the_year_in_synthetic_drugs.

Jenny Marder, "The Drug That Never Lets Go," PBS *Newshour*, September 20, 2012. www.pbs.org/newshour/multimedia/bath-salts.

Susan Newman, "Are 'Bath Salts' Just Hype?," *Psychology Today*, October 3, 2012. www.psychologytoday.com/blog/singletons/201210/are-bath-salts-just-hype.

Tony O'Neill, "The Truth Behind the Bath Salt 'Epidemic,'" *The Fix*, June 17, 2012. www.thefix.com/content/bath-salt-scare-10084?page=all.

Stephanie Pappas, "Latest Designer Drug Called 'Smiles' Linked to Teen Deaths," Fox News *Live Science*, September 24, 2012. www.foxnews.com/health/2012/09/24/latest-designer-drug-called-miles-linked-to-teen-deaths.

Eyder Peralta, "No 'Bath Salts' Drug Found in System of Face-Eating Attacker," *The Two-Way* (blog), blog, NPR, June 27, 2012. www.npr.org/blogs/thetwo-way/2012/06/27/155867335/no-bath-salts-drugs-found-in-system-of-face-eating-attacker.

Matthew Perrone, "After 'Bath Salts' Ban, Legal Ways to Get High Remain," *NBC News*, July 25, 2012. www.nbcnews.com/id/48317804/ns/health/t/after-bath-salts-ban-legal-ways-get-high-remain/#.UT9qq0rcu18.

Kent Sepkowitz, "What 'Bath Salts' Will—and Won't—Make You Do," *Daily Beast*, June 1, 2012. www.thedailybeast.com/articles/2012/06/01/what-bath-salts-will-and-won-t-make-you-do.html.

Natasha Vargas-Cooper, "Bath Salts: Deep in the Heart of America's New Drug Nightmare," *Spin*, June 14, 2012. www.spin.com/articles/bath lands-deep-heart-americas-new-drug-nightmare.

# Source Notes

## Overview

1. Quoted in CBS Connecticut, "Cops: Woman High on Bath Salts Wanted to 'Kill Someone and Eat Them,'" June 25, 2012. http://connecticut.cbslocal.com.
2. National Institute on Drug Abuse, "Bath Salts: An Emerging Danger," *Sara Bellum* (blog), February 5, 2013. http://teens.drugabuse.gov.
3. Substance Abuse and Mental Health Services Administration, "Will They Turn You into a Zombie? What Clinicians Need to Know About Synthetic Drugs," September 25, 2012. www.uclaisap.org.
4. Quoted in Nicole Brochu, "Synthetic Marijuana, Bath Salts Still Easily Obtained Despite Crackdown," *Sun Sentinel* (South FL), January 26, 2013. http://articles.sun-sentinel.com.
5. Quoted in Brochu, "Synthetic Marijuana, Bath Salts Still Easily Obtained Despite Crackdown."
6. Quoted in Tom Howell Jr., "D.C. Joins States on Synthetic Drug Ban," *Washington Times*, November 29, 2012. www.washingtontimes.com.
7. Quoted in Howell, "D.C. Joins States on Synthetic Drug Ban."
8. Quoted in Stephanie Pappas, "Latest Designer Drug Called 'Smiles' Linked to Teen Deaths," Fox News Live Science, September 24, 2012. www.foxnews.com.
9. Navy Alcohol and Drug Abuse Prevention, "Herbal Incense: An Awareness Presentation," 2010. www.public.navy.mil.
10. Michele M. Leonhart, "*Operation Log Jam* Press Conference," July 26, 2012. www.justice.gov.
11. National Institute on Drug Abuse, "Spice (Synthetic Marijuana)," December 2012. www.drugabuse.gov.
12. Quoted in Suzette Porter, "Effects of Synthetic Drugs Unknown," *TBN Weekly*, August 21, 2012. www.tbnweekly.com.
13. Quoted in Denise Mann, "Fake Marijuana Use Is a Serious Problem for Teens," WebMD, December 4, 2012. http://teens.webmd.com.
14. Quoted in Tammie Smith, "Drugs Known as 'Bath Salts' Pose Growing Danger," *Richmond* (VA) *Times-Dispatch*, July 8, 2012. www.timesdispatch.com.
15. Quoted in Matt McMillen, "'Bath Salts' Drug Trend: Expert Q & A," WebMD, February 26, 2013. www.webmd.com.

## How Serious a Problem Is Synthetic Drug Abuse?

16. Quoted in Michelle Hunter, "Clemson University Professor Created Synthetic Marijuana for Abuse Research," *New Orleanas Times-Picayune*, July 29, 2012. www.nola.com.
17. Quoted in David Zucchino, "Scientist's Research Produces a Dangerous High," *Los Angeles Times*, September 28, 2011. http://articles.latimes.com.
18. Quoted in Noelle Phillips, "Professor's 'Fake Weed' Now a Real Pain," *The State* (Columbia, SC), November 22, 2009. www.thestate.com.
19. Quoted in Zucchino, "Scientist's Research Produces a Dangerous High."
20. Quoted in Loreeta Canton, "AAPCC Issues Statement on the Synthetic Drug Abuse Prevention Act," American Association of Poison Control Centers, July 11, 2012. www.aapcc.org.

21. Quoted in Pam Louwagie, "Bath Salts Hit U.S. 'Like a Freight Train,'" *Minneapolis Star Tribune*, September 19, 2011. www.startribune.com.
22. Bertha K. Madras, "Designer Drugs: An Escalating Public Health Challenge," *Journal of Global Drug Policy and Practice*, September 10, 2012. www.globaldrugpolicy.org.
23. Quoted in Julie Scharper, "Cartoon Packaging May Hold Synthetic High, Real Danger," *Baltimore Sun*, September 14, 2012. http://articles.baltimoresun.com.
24. Quoted in Jennifer Van Pelt, "Synthetic Drugs—Fake Substances, Real Dangers," *Social Work Today*, July/August 2012. www.socialworktoday.com.
25. Lloyd D. Johnston et al., *Monitoring the Future: National Results on Drug Use*, February 2013. www.monitoringthefuture.org.
26. Johnston et al., *Monitoring the Future: National Results on Drug Use.*
27. Johnston et al., *Monitoring the Future: National Results on Drug Use.*
28. Carol L. Falkowski, "Drug Abuse Trends in Minneapolis/St. Paul, Minnesota: 2010," June 2011. www.dhs.state.mn.us.
29. Quoted in Chris Martinez, "Pasco Teen Hospitalized After Smoking Spice," ABC News, June 7, 2012. https://scripps.endplay.com.
30. Quoted in Fox News, "Synthetic Drug Use on the Rise," October 12, 2012. www.okc fox.com.

## What Are the Dangers of Synthetic Drugs?

31. Quoted in Sarah Horner, "Blaine Synthetic-Drug Overdose Case: Man Pleads Guilty in Friend's Death," *Pioneer Press* (St. Paul, MN), March 22, 2012. www.twincities.com.
32. Quoted in Pam Louwagie, "Blaine Party Survivors: 'All of Us Could Have Died That Night,'" *Minneapolis Star Tribune*, December 19, 2011. www.startribune.com.
33. Quoted in Louwagie, "Blaine Party Survivors."
34. Quoted in Anita Hassan, "Dangerous Designer Drug Hits the Streets," *Houston Chronicle*, September 23, 2012. www.chron.com.
35. Quoted in Jenny Marder, "The Drug That Never Lets Go," *PBS Newshour*, September 20, 2012. www.pbs.org.
36. Quoted in National Institute on Drug Abuse, "Spice: 'If You Use It, You're Experimenting on Yourself,'" *Sara Bellum* (blog), April 19, 2012. http://teens.drugabuse.gov.
37. Quoted in Nick Wasson, "Synthetic Pot Suspected in Kidney Failures," ABC News, February 14, 2013. http://abcnews.go.com.
38. Quoted in Jenifer Goodwin, "'Fake Marijuana' May Trigger Heart Trouble in Teens," *USA Today*, November 9, 2011. http://usatoday30.usatoday.com.
39. Quoted in Greg Allen, "Florida Bans Cocaine-Like 'Bath Salts' Sold in Stores," NPR, February 8, 2011. www.npr.org.
40. Quoted in Virginia Commonwealth University, "Dangerous Designer Drug Packs a One-Two Punch," March 14, 2013. www.cctr.vcu.edu.
41. Quoted in Bob Warren, "Snorting Bath Salts Pushed St. Tammany Man to Suicide," New Orleans *Times-Picayune*, January 16, 2011. www.nola.com.
42. Quoted in Warren, "Snorting Bath Salts Pushed St. Tammany Man to Suicide."
43. Quoted in Douglass Dowty, "What Syracuse Can Learn from Louisiana's 'Bath Salts' Epidemic," *Post-Standard* (Syracuse, NY), July 9, 2010. www.syracuse.com.

## How Should Synthetic Drugs Be Regulated?

44. Quoted in Marder, "The Drug That Never Lets Go."
45. Quoted in Marder, "The Drug That Never Lets Go."

46. Quoted in Jane Musgrave, "Eating Flesh 'Extremely Rare'; Experts Suspect Mix of Drugs," *Palm Beach Post*, May 30, 2012. www.palmbeachpost.com.

47. Quoted in Donna Leinwand Leger, "'Bath Salt' Poisonings Rise as Legislative Ban Tied Up," *USA Today*, April 12, 2012. http://usatoday30.usatoday.com.

48. Conforti and Turner, "Federal Law Attempts to Outlaw Synthetic Drugs," 2013. www.conforti-turner.com.

49. Quoted in Howard Owens, "From China White to Bath Salts, Designer Drugs Ongoing Public Safety Challenge," *Batavian* (Batavia, NY), July 24, 2012. http://thebatavian.com.

50. Quoted in Marder, "The Drug That Never Lets Go."

51. To the Maximus, "NEW Federal Synthetic Law!!! Sellers, [Manufacturers] and Distributors Are Going to Prison," July 10, 2012. http://tothemaximusblog.org.

52. To the Maximus, "NEW Federal Synthetic Law!!!"

53. Tad A. Nelson & Associates, "New Federal Ban on Bath Salts and Synthetic Marijuana in Effect in Texas," September 9, 2012. www.houstongalvestonlawyer.com.

54. Quoted in Larry Oakes, "Synthetic Drug Sales Booming on Web," *Minneapolis Star Tribune*, September 11, 2011. www.startribune.com.

55. Quoted in Oakes, "Synthetic Drug Sales Booming on Web."

56. Quoted in Ben Paynter, "The Big Business of Synthetic Highs," *Bloomberg Businessweek*, June 20, 2011. www.nbcnews.com.

## How Can Synthetic Drug Abuse Be Prevented?

57. Mike, Jan, and Daniel Rozga, "David's Story," K2 Drug Facts, July 2012. www.k2drugfacts.com.

58. Mike, Jan, and Daniel Rozga, "David's Story."

59. Mike Rozga, "The Dangers of Synthetic Cannabinoids and Stimulants," Senate Caucus on International Narcotics Control, April 6, 2011. www.drugcaucus.senate.gov.

60. Mike, Jan, and Daniel Rozga, "Advocates for Action Guest Post: Turning Tragedy into Purpose," Office of National Drug Control Policy, White House, October 19, 2012. www.whitehouse.gov.

61. Quoted in Madison Mathews, "School Program Tackles Synthetic Drug Issue," *Johnson City (TN) Press*, March 14, 2012. www.johnsoncitypress.com.

62. Quoted in Mathews "School Program Tackles Synthetic Drug Issue."

63. Quoted in Paul Kampe, "Judge Educates Clarkston Parents, Teenagers on Synthetic Drug K2/Spice," *Oakland Press*, October 4, 2012. www.theoaklandpress.com.

64. Quoted in WJLE Radio, "District Attorney Randy York Announces New Anti-Drug Campaign," October 17, 2012. www.wjle.com.

65. Nancy Barnes, "Star Tribune Editor: Synthetic-Drug Dangers Are Under Our Spotlight," *Minneapolis Star Tribune*, January 14, 2012. www.startribune.com.

66. Barnes, "Star Tribune Editor: Synthetic-Drug Dangers Are Under Our Spotlight."

67. Barnes, "Star Tribune Editor: Synthetic-Drug Dangers Are Under Our Spotlight."

68. Barnes, "Star Tribune Editor: Synthetic-Drug Dangers Are Under Our Spotlight."

69. Mike, Jan, and Daniel Rozga, "Advocates for Action Guest Post: Turning Tragedy into Purpose."

# List of Illustrations

# Index

Note: Boldface page numbers indicate illustrations.

# About the Author

Peggy J. Parks holds a bachelor of science degree from Aquinas College in Grand Rapids, Michigan, where she graduated magna cum laude. An author who has written more than a hundred educational books for children and young adults, Parks lives in Muskegon, Michigan, a town that she says inspires her writing because of its location on the shores of Lake Michigan.